THE COMPLETE PERIMENOPAUSE WEIGHT LOSS PLAN

A SIMPLE 27 DAY PROGRAM TO HELP YOU MANAGE
HORMONAL WEIGHT GAIN, FLATTEN YOUR BELLY
AND BOOST SLUGGISH METABOLISM

SARAH HILL

CONTENTS

Thank you so much for purchasing this book!

Scan the QR code or visit our webpage via the link below to receive a FREE mini e-book:

"7 EASY STEPS to Reduce Hormonal Bloating Fast

+

5 Day Quick Fix Meal Plan"

www.perimenopausematters.com

INTRODUCTION

Don't regret growing older. It is a privilege denied to many.

— *UNKNOWN*

Getting older is an inevitable part of life, but the changes that come with it aren't always what we expect. Going through perimenopause can be a confusing experience. It can feel as though you are disoriented in your own body with the onset of hormonal ups and downs. It can even leave you feeling isolated and alone in your struggles to reclaim some semblance of the normality you knew when you were younger.

The good news is that you're not alone. Some women experience perimenopause more mildly than others. If you're not one of those lucky women, you're in good company with millions of women around the world. It's a sisterhood of hormonal upheavals, and many women are just as confused as you are about why their bodies are turning traitor on them despite their best efforts.

One of the biggest hormonal culprits in a woman's life is estrogen. It takes hold and turns your life upside down when you hit puberty, and it does it all over again when you make your way toward menopause. It's a vital hormone, but that doesn't make the chaos it can wreak an easier pill to swallow. What does help, though, is having knowledge on your side. When you have a better understanding of what's really going on in your body, you can deal with it more easily and find your way around the obstacles you face.

The same thing happened to me, and I was caught completely off guard. I felt bewildered and betrayed by my own body. After all, I had always been a woman of average size despite my bad habit of chronic yo-yo dieting—which I now know was one of the worst things I could have done for my health. I had also always labored under the misconception that your genetics were solely responsible for how your weight changed as you got older. Along with that, I believed periods and moodiness were inextricably linked and pregnancy meant gaining loads of weight. In fact, that is exactly what I experienced, so, in essence, my assumptions were self-fulfilling prophecies; why would I ever believe differently if I didn't know any different?

By the time I had gone through my third pregnancy and given birth to a beautiful baby, I gained tons of weight. I kind of shrugged my shoulders and thought that was it: My life was over. Perimenopause was just beginning for me, and the first symptoms were setting in. I was experiencing sweats, blurry vision, tiredness, and brain fog. I also have three kids… you do the math.

Then, something extraordinary happened. At the age of 37, I caught a glimpse of myself in the mirror. I was faced with the reality of my situation when my saggy butt and flabby belly pouch stared back at me.

It's tempting to shy away from the mirror and resign yourself to the middle-aged spread, and of course, I had the option to do just that, but that's not what I wanted for my life. I woke up one day and decided it would not beat me!

I was unhappy; I wanted to take back control over my body; and I started researching nutrition, exercise, and muscle-building techniques. I was determined to make the changes that would give me the results I wanted.

I understand how frustrating it is when your body changes without your knowledge or permission thereof. The first time you realize it is when things don't add up anymore, the symptoms start appearing, and the number on the scale begins creeping up. Suddenly, the old tricks do not work. Even when you do not change anything, the pounds keep piling up. The weight accumulates around your belly and thighs. You just keep thinking: What the heck am I doing wrong? That's what happened to me and what happens to millions of women around the world. The silver lining is that you can turn things around and take control of your life, and I'm here to show you how to do it.

The key to successful and sustainable weight loss in perimenopause is, very simply, a change in eating habits. That is it. 70% of success in losing the unwanted pounds is simply sticking to a nutritious, wholesome diet, on a long term basis. If you add the remaining 30% , which is movement, sleep and stressing less - you have the recipe for achieving your goals even quicker.

This is why the main focus of this book is planning your weight loss journey, when your body is going through a storm of hormones, and a metabolic shift happens as a result. Some, or all parts of our diet will need looking at, and most likely, require changing or tweaking a little bit. Success is guaranteed if you simply follow it through.

In this book, you will discover:

- What perimenopause is
- The symptoms
- Why you are prone to gaining weight as you get older
- Why managing your weight is increasingly important as you age
- How to mentally prepare for lifestyle changes

- How to track your symptoms and why it matters
- How to calculate and track your calories
- Why setting SMART goals is important and how to do it
- How to measure your progress and why it's important
- Delicious, healthy recipes and an easy-to-follow meal plan to help you kick-start your physical, mental, and emotional transformation
- In 27 days, you really can lose up to 10 pounds in weight, flatten your belly, and feel so much better despite experiencing symptoms of perimenopause. All the tools and knowledge to help you achieve that are in this book.

It took some time to learn everything I needed to know and put it into practice, but slowly—very, very slowly—it all came together. When this happened, I started seeing massive results. Most of my peri-menopausal symptoms lessened or disappeared due to simple diet adjustments. I've brought all of that knowledge together to help you and the millions of other women who have been caught off guard by perimenopause just like I was. If you're ready to transform your body and your life, sit tight and keep reading; I'm going to help teach you everything you need to know to reclaim control and win back your happiness.

WELCOME TO PERIMENOPAUSE

Perimenopause is a natural part of any woman's life as she gets older, but the fact that it's normal doesn't make it any less of a pain to deal with. What does make perimenopause more manageable is knowledge. That's why I'm going to take you through everything you could possibly need to know to navigate your way through this time of change and come out on the other side sane and healthy.

WHAT EXACTLY IS PERIMENOPAUSE?

Pretty much every woman has heard of and knows of the big M: menopause. However, not too many women have heard of or know about peri-menopause. Most people associate the signs of perimenopause as being menopausal because the timeline between perimenopause, menopause, and postmenopause is literally only 12 months. However, the symptoms of this overall great hormonal and transitional roller coaster may be felt for years. Here's how it works.

Hormonal changes start happening in your body as you start getting along in age, and you may notice changes in your body and menstrual cycle as well. This is perimenopause: It is the transition period between the period where you are a fertile woman and menopause. It's a time of great change. These changes affect each woman differently because every woman's body is different, so you can never take another woman's experience as a reference for what your experience will be like.

The symptoms most women associate with menopause come from perimenopause because it's during this time that your hormones are completely scrambled due to the changes happening. You will still experience symptoms during menopause which normally fade away once you have completely stopped menstruating and have entered post-menopause.

Perimenopause generally starts in a woman's 40s. However, perimenopause can begin as early as in her 30s. On average, perimenopause sets in only a couple of years up to 10 years before menopause, lasting an average of four years, but it could also only take a few months or last longer. It's an incredibly (and hormonally) turbulent time in a woman's life. It's not unlike going through puberty as a teenager, but the reasons for these hormonal ups and downs are vastly different.

So why do we go through perimenopause? What makes it happen? This internal game of hormonal Twister starts when your ovaries begin acting up in preparation for a final shutdown when they completely stop releasing eggs. Natural curiosity might lead you to question why your body would need to stop releasing eggs in the first place. The answer is twofold.

Women are born with all of their eggs already formed inside of them. Unlike men, who produce new sperm every few days, women don't make eggs. They are simply released once a month. This means your eggs are aging just like the rest of your body. If an older egg were to be fertilized, there is a much bigger risk of something going wrong with the baby.

A woman's ability to physically carry a baby to full term decreases as she gets older. Her body isn't as capable as when she was younger, and this could lead to difficulties and complications which could hurt both mom and baby if an older woman falls pregnant.

Now, this isn't to say an older woman can't enjoy a safe, healthy pregnancy and deliver a perfectly healthy baby. It just means that the risk is higher, and the complications are greater.

PERIMENOPAUSE SYMPTOMS

You don't necessarily have to go to a doctor to be able to tell whether you are in perimenopause or not; most women can observe their bodies and come to the conclusion themselves. Let's discuss the signs and symptoms of perimenopause, so you know exactly what you're keeping an eye out for.

It's important to bear in mind that every woman experiences perimenopause differently. Some women barely notice any changes in their bodies or symptoms; others aren't so lucky, and the symptoms can make them downright miserable. Whether you experience mild or stronger symptoms, arming yourself with knowledge will help you figure your way through the journey more easily.

The First Signs

The very first signs of perimenopause relate to your menstrual cycle. You may notice your monthly cycle isn't quite what you're used to. You could start noticing irregularities such as your period starting up earlier or later than usual. For instance, if you have a regular 28-day cycle, it may end up being a 21-day or 35-day cycle sometimes. You may even notice you've skipped a month altogether, and your next period is heavier than normal. If you aren't a woman with a menstrual cycle that's as regular as clockwork, it may be a little more difficult to pick up on these first signs unless you suddenly start skipping a period here and there.

The Symptoms Explained

The symptoms of perimenopause happen because your body is essentially going through an estrogen withdrawal, as your ovaries start producing less of it heading toward menopause. We often say estrogen, but it should be estrogens because there are different kinds of estrogen produced. Since puberty, your body has been depending on estrogen for a variety of reasons. It affects the following:

- How your menstrual cycle is regulated
- Your reproductive organs (including vaginal lubrication)
- Your urinary tract
- Skin
- Hair
- Bones
- Breasts
- Brain
- Cardiovascular system
- Pelvic muscles

Considering all these systems and organs being influenced by estrogen, it's no wonder your body goes into a bit of a crisis when the levels start dropping drastically.

▷ **Hot Flashes**

This is probably the single-most infamous symptom of hormonal change in a woman. During a hot flash, you feel like you are overheating and you might even get a little (or a lot) sweaty. These episodes normally last for roughly 10 minutes, and about 35%–50% of women going through perimenopause have hot flashes ("Perimenopause: Rocky road to menopause," 2020).

These flashes can happen during the night or day but more often occur at night. Your average hot flash starts in your upper body—generally, your chest, neck, face, or the top of your head—and can vary from feeling warm to feeling like your body has become your own personal sauna. While these overheating episodes can last up to 10 years after menopause in up to 10% of women, there is a silver lining. The good news is that hot flashes often decrease and disappear altogether within a year or two of entering postmenopause ("Perimenopause: Rocky road to menopause," 2020).

▷ **Mood Swings**

Another notorious symptom of perimenopause is mood fluctuation. Despite it being one of the most joked-about and clichéd symptoms of perimenopause, it only has a disruptive effect on about 10%–20% of perimenopausal women. It's also important to remember that if you do experience mood swings, they could be anywhere from mild to moderate depending on how your body handles the change in hormones ("Perimenopause: Rocky road to menopause," 2020).

It's crucial to understand that perimenopause isn't likely to cause you to become depressed, anxious, or suffer permanent grumpiness.

- **Tip:** Getting regular exercise; eating a diet rich in whole grains and complex carbohydrates; and cutting back on refined sugar helps stabilize your blood sugar. Blood sugar ups and downs are known for making people "hangry" which could be contributing to your moodiness. Ditching refined sugar and upping your exercise routine can improve your blood sugar and insulin response to prevent the highs and lows that send your family running for cover. A healthy diet and regular exercise are recommended for reducing hot flashes.

▷ **Problems Sleeping**

Changes in your sleep cycle are a normal part of getting older, so pinning your sleep disturbances solely on perimenopause isn't quite fair. However, it could be a contributing factor for those sleep problems and even night sweats. About 40% of women going through perimenopause experience changes or difficulties with their sleeping cycles, but it's useful to know that insomnia is a common complaint among both men and women as they age ("Perimenopause: Rocky road to menopause," 2020).

- **Tip:** To combat sleep difficulties, try maintaining a routine, reducing your caffeine intake, and only using your bed for sleep. Following a healthy diet that is rich in whole grains and fresh fruits and vegetables may help reduce night sweats. Also, doing some yoga may help you relax for a better night's sleep.

▷ **Period Bleeding**

As I've said before, changes in your period are a normal part of perimenopause. However, even if you don't experience a change in the length of your cycle or skipping a month altogether, you could experience a change in how much you bleed. Estrogen isn't the only hormone that fluctuates and decreases during this time. Progesterone also decreases.

Progesterone is responsible for regulating the growth of your womb's lining which is the part you bleed out during menstruation. You might experience that lining growing thicker than normal which results in heavier bleeding.

You may also experience increased discomfort and difficulties if you have endometriosis (when tissues similar to the tissue lining the inside of your womb start growing outside the womb) or fibroids (uncomfortable but not harmful growths on the inside walls of your womb).

- **Tip:** Contraceptives may help boost hormone levels to help even them out. However, if you don't want to go a medical route, understanding hormone fluctuations makes this in-between bleeding slightly less stressful. In this situation, preparedness by keeping feminine products on hand at all times and moving away from wearing white pants can also lessen the stress of it all.

▷ **Vaginal Lubrication Problems**

Estrogen is responsible for keeping your vaginal walls thick, lubricated, and elastic. When your levels of estrogen fall drastically, the impact may be felt in vaginal dryness and thinner or less flexible than before. These changes could be a contributing factor to waning libido, as they could lead to uncomfortable or even painful sex with a partner.

- **Tip:** There are estrogen creams and vaginal moisturizers available on the market. However, if you want a more natural approach, go easy on the feminine and other hygiene products. These products can upset the delicate pH and bacterial balance to keep it clean and healthy all by itself. Hygiene products can dry and upset that delicate balance. Another way to combat loss of vaginal tissue elasticity is to enjoy an active sex life. If sex is uncomfortable, try adding some lubricant to make it more comfortable.

▷ **Cognitive Changes**

Estrogen and progesterone have a hand in how your brain functions. Then again, so does aging in general because both men and women have the same complaints about decreasing brain function. Aging and hormonal changes combined could leave you

finding it difficult to concentrate and even having
some short-term memory issues.

- **Tip:** Include omega-3 fatty acids in your diet
  and get regular exercise to help boost brain
  function. You can also try some fun brain-
  training games and puzzles to keep your
  mental muscle flexed.

▷ **Bone Density Loss**

This is a very real concern and often has a devas-
tating impact on women as they grow older. In
Chapter 2, I discuss this in more detail, as this is a
critical concern that women should address before
bone density starts to decrease.

Fear tries to get us to give up, but faith takes us all the way to victory.

— JOYCE MEYER

PERIMENOPAUSE, MENOPAUSE, AND YOUR WEIGHT

Menopause has four distinct stages. Perimenopause is one of the stages, and it's the one that is the most impactful for a woman. Let's explore the different stages of menopause. I also want to tell you how and why perimenopause may cause weight changes.

THE FOUR STAGES OF MENOPAUSE

I've just told you that menopause is made up of four stages. Considering the changes you experience along the way and how they affect your body and your life, it can be scary to realize it isn't just one stage and then it's over. Though four stages seems like a lot, don't fret. Just because there are four stages doesn't mean things are four times as bad. It's only one stage that causes the most hassle for women: perimenopause.

Premenopause

The word premenopause gives you an idea of what it means. "Pre" means before. It refers to the entire stage of your reproductive life before menopause. This stage begins when you first start menstruating at puberty and continues until you have your very last period which marks the end of menopause. This stage of your life normally lasts 30–40 years.

Perimenopause

The "peri" part of perimenopause means around or about, so perimenopause means "around menopause." As I've explained, it is the time of hormonal change that happens as your ovaries and body start producing less estrogen and progesterone. During this time, you are likely to experience at least some of the symptoms listed above to some degree, whether mild or more intense. Perimenopause falls under premenopause because you still menstruate during perimenopause, and you have only gone through menopause once you haven't had a period for 12 months.

Menopause

Menopause itself lasts only 12 months and typically occurs around 45–55 years of age with the average age being 51. This is the time when your ovaries have stopped producing ova or eggs, and the majority of estrogen production has also stopped. Menopause is marked by having no menstrual cycle for 12 months. If you have a period at any time within 12 months, even 11 months apart, you aren't in menopause yet. You are still in perimenopause.

Important Note: Once you haven't menstruated for a year or more, you aren't likely to bleed again. However, if you do experience vaginal bleeding or a period once you have entered menopause or post-menopause, it's not normal and you should immediately consult your doctor. Vaginal bleeding after menopause could be caused by several reasons. Various reasons are harmless, but there are a few potential reasons which have some serious health implications. The reasons for postmenopausal bleeding include the following:

- Bleeding from your rectum or urinary tract
- Cancer in your womb including uterine sarcoma and endometrial cancer

- Cervical or vaginal cancer
- Endometrial atrophy when the lining of your womb becomes thin
- Endometrial hyperplasia is when the lining of your womb is growing excessively.
- Endometriosis is an infection of the lining of your womb.
- Fibroids in your womb
- Polyps in your womb
- Some medications like tamoxifen and hormone replacement therapy
- Trauma to your pelvis
- Vaginal atrophy can happen when the lining of your vagina becomes thin.

Postmenopause

The part of the part "post" means after, so it means "after menopause." Once you have spent those 12 months of no period for menopause, you will enter the rest of your menstruation-free life. This is when you are postmenopausal. However, as I've just mentioned, if you experience any bleeding after you have gone through menopause, you should consult your doctor to make sure it's not a harmful health condition.

Important Notes: The symptoms women usually associate with menopause are generally at their worst during perimenopause. These symptoms should lessen and go away once you have reached and gone through menopause. However, some women have reported their symptoms getting worse in that first year or two after they have gone through the 12 months of menopause.

Just because you have stopped menstruating doesn't mean you have necessarily come to the end of hormonal changes. There are natural hormonal changes that happen as you age, and therefore, it is possible to still experience hormonal shifts in post-menopause.

PERIMENOPAUSE AND WEIGHT GAIN

Needless to say, hot flashes and moodiness are two really annoying aspects of going through the whole menopause process. Does nature have to get on your last perimenopausal nerve by bringing on the middle-aged spread as well? I can hear the mental groan that just happened in your head. Trust me: There are a lot of other women out there groaning about having to deal with the same thing as they get along in years. I'm here to tell you how to combat that unwanted weight gain being egged on by your hormones. However, before we can get to that part, I need to help you understand why it's happening. There is nothing more frustrating than struggling with a problem and not knowing why it's happening in the first place. How are you supposed to know how to overcome an obstacle if you don't know why it's happening? Right, let's dive into the reasons you gain weight as you get older and go through perimenopause.

Interesting to Know: The average amount of weight a woman gains during perimenopause is five pounds with only about 20% of women gaining up to 10 pounds (Hosterman, 2015).

Why Weight Gain Happens

Let me start by saying this: It's not all hormonal. Yes, hormones play their fair part in the process, but they're not solely to blame. The truth of the matter is that weight gain is associated with getting older for a variety of reasons. The good news is you can control your diet and lifestyle to minimize the impact of these natural bodily changes on your health and weight.

The reason for age-related weight gain is metabolism. It all comes down to your metabolism, but the answer isn't quite as cut-and-dried as that. Why does your metabolism tend to slow down as you get older?

▷ **Hormones**

Yes, hormonal changes form part of the metabolic slowdown puzzle. There are two possible reasons your weight may fluctuate or go up as you get older. Estrogen plays a big role in controlling your metabolism and regulating insulin. If you have too much or too little of it, you're going to feel the side effects.

When you first enter perimenopause, there is a communication disconnect between your ovaries, pituitary gland, and a part of your brain called the hypothalamus. This "loose connection" in your body's communication between its different parts causes your estrogen levels to fluctuate, and sometimes, that fluctuation can be quite wild. When this happens, you could end up having too much estrogen in your body. Let's just clear something up quickly. I'm not saying that having a little more estrogen than normal will make you fat. What I am saying is that you could gain weight if you have a very high level of estrogen. The cells that produce insulin may become irritated when you have too much estrogen in your body, and you may not be producing enough insulin to regulate your blood sugar—thereby increasing your risk of weight gain.

On the flip side of the coin, estrogen levels do decline as you make your way toward menopause. It's one of those inevitabilities, so your levels will drop over time even if you experience fluctuations and possibly raised estrogen levels earlier on in peri-menopause as I just mentioned. There is a specific type of estrogen called estradiol which helps out with regulating your metabolism. When levels of estradiol drop, your metabolism isn't regulated as well as it used to be, and that can lead to weight gain.

There is yet another reason low levels of estrogen may cause weight gain. Your ovaries are the primary sources, but they aren't the only ones responsible for producing estrogen. Other sources include your adrenal glands and body fat. Yes, you read that right. Body fat produces a small amount of estrogen, and in the absence of ovary-supplied estrogen, your body is going to get it from wherever it can. Your body bumps up its fat-storing to increase your body fat by stockpiling all extra energy into fat.

Interesting to Know: When you are younger, you are more likely to store body fat in your hips, thighs, and breasts. When estrogen levels drop, your body tends to start storing fat around your midsection. Why? Your body begins to store more abdominal fat, also called visceral fat. This is the type of fat that is stored inside your body around your internal organs as opposed to subcutaneous fat stored underneath your skin.

▷ **Muscle Loss**

Age-related muscle loss is called sarcopenia, and it affects both men and women. Did you know that you can lose up to 3–5% of your lean muscle mass every decade after you turn 30 ("Preserve your muscle mass," 2016)? It may not sound like much, but decreasing your muscle mass by 15% between the ages of 30 and 60 has a huge impact on your life. Not only does it create a weakness that places strain on your bones and causes mobility issues but it also slows your metabolism down. Lean muscle requires fuel to build and maintain. The more muscle you have, the more calories you need per day to keep your body going. Losing muscle decreases the number of calories you burn daily—slowing your metabolism down.

One possible contributing factor to losing muscle as you get older is a decline in testosterone. Estrogen is seen as the female hormone while testosterone is viewed as the male hormone. Labeling these hormones as male or female doesn't mean men and women don't have both in their bodies. Women just have more estrogen, and men have more testosterone. Testosterone is not only associated with libido but also with your body's muscle-building capabilities. As you age, testosterone is another hormone that drops and so does your ability to build and maintain muscle.

▷ **Hunger, Appetite, and Calories**

We've just gone through how lower estrogen levels can slow your metabolism down and how muscle loss slows your metabolism down. Lower estrogen levels also mess with how two other hormones function: leptin and neuropeptide Y. These two hormones regulate how full you feel after meals and your appetite. When they don't work properly, you could find yourself feeling less satisfied after meals and hungrier in general which could see you eating more than you should. To make matters worse, you need to eat fewer calories as you get older because of muscle loss and a slower metabolism, so feeling hungrier and less full after meals is like adding fuel to the weight gain fire.

WHY WEIGHT MANAGEMENT IS SO IMPORTANT

Some women may think that weight loss and maintaining a healthy weight throughout perimenopause and beyond is an impossible task. You may find friends, family, or acquaintances resigning themselves to middle-aged weight gain and not worrying about it or trying to control it. The reality is that weight loss and maintenance are challenges as you get older. Perimenopause is part of the aging process, and aging generally makes many aspects of life more challenging. However, you need to keep your chin up and understand that it may not be as easy as when you were in your 20s, but it's not impossible.

Many women dread perimenopausal weight gain because we live in a society that is body-image-focused. However, there is more reason to want to keep the pounds off than just fitting into your jeans. Maintaining a healthy weight throughout your life is vital for your health.

Healthy Aging

There are various aspects of your body and health that are affected by getting older. Your risk of a variety of health concerns increases, including the following:

- High cholesterol
- Heart disease (cardiovascular disease)
- High blood pressure (hypertension)
- Metabolic syndrome (having high cholesterol, high blood pressure, high blood sugar, and being overweight all at once)
- Osteoarthritis (deterioration of the bone and cartilage in joints causing inflammation)
- Osteoporosis ("brittle bone" disease)
- Stroke (cerebrovascular disease)
- Type 2 diabetes (high blood sugar)

Other health conditions increase in risk as you get older. However, the ones listed above have one thing in common. The risk further increases with carrying around more pounds than you should. By actively losing some weight and working to maintain a healthy weight, you can reduce your risk of developing every one of these conditions, so maintaining a healthy weight helps you live a long, happy, and healthy life.

Abdominal Fat

Remember I mentioned visceral and subcutaneous fat a few paragraphs ago? Well, why does it matter which type of fat you have? Fat under your skin comes with a health price as it is. You are going to be at a higher risk for health conditions, but it's not as dangerous as abdominal fat.

Everybody has to have some abdominal fat; it's meant to cushion your internal organs and keep them where they are. The problem starts when you have too much abdominal fat. This type of fat prompts your body to produce hormones and proteins that create inflammation in cells and tissues. This inflammation can damage internal organs and arteries which leads to further complications like heart disease.

Going through perimenopause, your body shifts from storing fat under the skin to inside your abdominal cavity, increasing the amount of visceral fat. Losing weight and controlling how much abdominal fat you have reduces your risk of developing potentially life-threatening diseases.

HEALTHY DIET AND LIFESTYLE

I've just explained why you're likely to gain weight during perimenopause, but why is it so hard to lose that weight? Many of the things that make it easier to gain weight double up as reasons it's so hard to drop it again. Mother Nature is not playing ball with women's aging bodies, is she? Well, the good news is I'm here to help.

I cannot stress enough that living a healthy lifestyle and eating a healthy diet are your best chances at losing weight and keeping it off during the various stages of menopause. This can seem like a challenge as you get older—after all, you have less energy and stamina; you're naturally inclined to become less active; and you may be feeling the effects of some past injuries. There are many reasons why keeping up an active lifestyle as you get older seems to be more challenging. Following a healthy diet can seem equally as challenging—even in your youth—because our modern society covets processed foods packed with empty calories without much nutritional value.

The first step to restructuring your life is to figure out what your daily caloric needs are and how much exercise you should be getting. I'm going to provide you with the formulas for working out your daily calorie needs in a later chapter. For now, let's ask the question, "How much exercise do I actually need?"

According to the Centers for Disease Control and Prevention (CDC), this is how much and what types of exercise you should be getting per week ("How much physical activity do adults need?", 2020):

- Moderate intensity cardio/aerobic exercise: 150 minutes per week
- Vigorous-intensity cardio/aerobic exercise: 75 minutes per week
- Combination of moderate and vigorous-intensity cardio/aerobic exercise: two or more days weekly
- Strength or resistance training exercise to build muscle: two or more days weekly

Moderate Intensity Test: Use a talk test to tell whether you are working out at a low or moderate intensity. Talk to a friend or have a conversation with yourself while you are exercising. If you can comfortably hold a conversation, you're working out at a low intensity. If you can have a breathy conversation (speaking a few words between breaths), you are working out at a moderate intensity.

If you are going through perimenopause at the average age of your 40s and you are not used to getting regular cardio exercise, it's probably best to start slower. Try to aim for 150 minutes of moderate cardio per week. That's as little as 30 minutes of cardio per day across five days per week.

Did You Know?: Walking is a fantastic form of exercise that gets your body moving and your heart working. You may need to walk briskly for double the amount of time you would need to jog to burn the same number of calories, but the holistic health payoffs are similar.

What are the benefits of regular exercise as you get older?

- You stay flexible, and you maintain the range of motion in your joints and limbs.
- You keep your bones strong and healthy—this is especially important, as decreasing levels of estrogen can cause bone density loss.
- You maintain your sense of balance to prevent falls and injury.
- Exercise burns energy, but it also increases your energy level over time.

- Your muscles are working, so, providing your diet is nutrient-dense, you're working on building and preserving lean muscle mass.
- You're keeping your heart and lungs healthy.

Calorie Deficit: Caution

It's become such general knowledge in the diet world that it's turned into a cliché. To lose weight, calories taken in must be less than calories out, or you need to take in fewer calories than you burn as energy. Now, I will be giving you a rundown of how to calculate your daily caloric needs in Chapter 6, but right now, I want to explain and caution you about creating a calorie deficit.

Yes, a calorie deficit is needed for weight loss, but creating too much of a deficit can be really bad for your health—especially when you're not a spring chicken anymore. One of the most infamous ways women lose weight is by crash dieting. They drastically slash their calories for a relatively short time to drop lots of weight as quickly as possible. The problem with this is that the moment they start eating normally again, the weight just piles back on, and often, they gain more weight back than they lost.

It's just a really bad idea. Nobody should be crash dieting, irrespective of their age. Please don't do this. It's so unhealthy and not sustainable. As a middle-aged woman, the dangers of cutting your calories too much include the following:

▷ **Malnutrition**

You don't have to be starving to death to be malnourished. In fact, you can be overweight and still be malnourished. Malnourishment doesn't mean you aren't eating enough; it means you aren't getting in enough essential nutrients for your body to stay healthy. You can be eating an excess of empty calories in unhealthy, processed foods but taking in very little proper nutrition. However, you're bound to become malnourished if you don't eat enough.

Provided you are eating a healthy, balanced diet including a wide variety of produce, you need to eat a bare minimum of 1,200 calories per day. Don't take that as a suggestion because it's not. I'm just telling you what the absolute bare minimum is and that's only if you are eating lots of varied whole foods that are packed with vitamins and minerals.

▷ Slowed Metabolism

There's a myth that cutting calories will slow your metabolism down or even put your body into starvation mode. No, a modest calorie restriction will not slow your metabolism down. However, slashing your calories too much is likely to do just that. Your metabolism slows down because your body doesn't have enough energy to burn to stay healthy and function properly. When it doesn't have sufficient energy to burn, your body interprets the situation as if there is a famine, and it starts switching off or slowing down nonessential functions to conserve energy. A modest calorie restriction, however, provides your body with enough energy to be healthy but less than it needs to maintain your current weight.

▷ Estrogen Production Reduction

As a perimenopausal woman, your estrogen production is already on the decline and causing symptoms. Why would you want to do something that will actively reduce your estrogen levels even further? When you eat too few calories and your body starts slowing down your metabolism, one of the functions it slows down is reproductive hormones. After all, having a baby isn't essential or ideal when your body thinks there's a food shortage. You might know you're just depriving your body of calories to lose weight, but it hasn't got a clue what's going on and naturally assumes there isn't food around.

▷ Bone Density Loss

One of the reasons women suffer from a loss of bone density as they get older is a decline in estrogen. You might be saying to yourself, "Estrogen is a sex hormone; what does it have to do with my bones?" I mentioned that estrogens play a part in a variety of different bodily functions. One of these functions is to make sure the cells that make your bones, called osteoblasts, work properly. These osteoblasts don't make bone as efficiently when your estrogen level drops.

Your bones are living tissues. Your body reabsorbs old bone cells and replaces them with new ones all the time. Estrogen slows down this bone cell turnover and promotes the formation of new bone cells. As you get older, your body produces less estrogen, and your body also experiences difficulties absorbing enough of the vitamins and minerals essential for bone growth.

Eating too little reduces your estrogen levels further and also doesn't allow you to eat enough to take in as much of the vitamins and minerals you need for healthy bone formation. You could be setting yourself down the path of developing osteoporosis by weakening your bones.

▷ Immunity

Your immune system depends on the vitamins and minerals from your food to remain fighting fit in the face of illness and injury. You are making yourself vulnerable to disease and slow injury healing when you're not eating enough and giving your body the nutrients it needs to keep your immune system running in perfect shape.

▷ Muscle Loss

I've explained that you inevitably lose some muscle mass as you get older. Not eating enough will make you lose even more muscle. Building muscle isn't an essential function in the face of famine and hard times, so your body puts that on the back burner. Did you know if your calorie intake is too low for too long and your body isn't getting enough energy to function, it starts what is called catabolism? It starts cannibalizing itself by reabsorbing muscle tissue for energy. Unless you have a history or are dealing with certain serious eating disorders, that's not going to happen, but slashing your calories too low tells your body to stop wasting precious energy on healthy muscle growth and maintenance.

If you really want to do something, you will find a way. If you don't, you will find an excuse.

— JIM ROHN

3

PREPARING FOR A HEALTHY DIET: DAY 1

The next 27 days will reshape your body for a happier and healthier you. In the next few chapters I'm going to take you through preparing for weight loss and a new healthy lifestyle. After that we're going to get right into a 21-day weight loss plan. These first five days of preparation for your weight loss and health transformation are crucial to keeping you on track and making your new habits stick in the long run. This preparation process involves self-reflection and identifying areas of your life which need changing as well as ways to track your progress and stay motivated.

This chapter is dedicated to the first phase of preparing yourself to adopt a healthier diet. Changing your diet and restricting your calories, even modestly, can be a challenge. People are naturally creatures of habit. We like to hold on to habits that feel comfortable, and the discomfort of change opens the door to falling right back into the habits we're trying to change.

It's exactly because of this tendency to hold on or fall back on comfortable habits that you need to prepare for making your move toward a healthier diet and weight loss. Sure, you can just decide to eat healthier, but without proper preparation, you're just making it harder than it has to be. So you've decided to change your diet; now, it's time to take a step back and start preparing. With this meal plan I've created, you'll have 27 days to work on it. This includes five days to prepare for what's ahead, 21 days of the meal plan, and the one final day to review your overall progress.

By all means, extend the first five days, if you need to. It might take you longer to self-reflect, observe your symptoms and properly get into the mindset of change. That is absolutely okay! Observing yourself on this journey is a crucial step to success, do not skip it! Anyone can diet for a few days or weeks, not everyone manages to actually change their lifestyle. These steps are here to set you up for success.

▷ Keep It Safe

I'm providing you with all the knowledge, structure, and tools you need to combat the middle-aged spread and keep the weight off. What I'm telling you is based on research and personal experience, but I am not a medical professional or dietician.

It is vitally important that you seek advice and all clear from your physician before you attempt any lifestyle or dietary changes that affect your health. This is especially important if you have any preexisting health conditions. What if you don't have any health conditions that you know of? Still, go see your doctor. You never know if you may have any underlying health conditions that haven't made their presence felt.

A qualified medical doctor is the only person who can give you a physical exam and the green light to go ahead with the changes you want to make. Your doctor might even be able to give you further advice or make recommendations for the changes you want to make.

The Bottom Line: Go see your doctor before making any dietary or lifestyle changes. Your health and safety are worth the trip and the exam.

▷ **Change Your Attitude**

Weight loss isn't just a physical experience: It's just as much a mental experience. You need to mentally prepare to take on this challenge. Simply deciding to lose weight isn't going to get you there.

According to Pamela Peeke (2007), MD, the author of *Fit to Live*, you must "cut the mental fat, and that will lead to cutting the waistline fat."

What she's saying is you need to think yourself thin, and your body will follow. What does thinking yourself thin mean? What mindset do you have to adopt to be successful at adopting and sticking to a new way of healthy eating?

▷ **Have Patience**

We live in a world of instant gratification. If we want something, we want it right now. Think about instant messaging. How often do you text someone with a question only to find waiting for an answer one of the most frustrating things in the world? I bet sitting and watching your phone waiting for that notification to pop up is like watching paint dry!

More often than not, weight gain doesn't happen overnight—it's usually a gradual process. If it's taken you months or even years to gain the weight, you can't expect it to drop off overnight or even in a week. Losing weight the healthy way takes time. That's not to say it has to take you months or years to lose it again. I'm just pointing out that when you're on a journey of healthy, sustainable weight loss, you aren't going to wake up in a week, and the weight is miraculously gone. A realistic and healthy rate of weight loss is one to two pounds per week. At that rate, you are not trying to lose too much too quickly, and the efforts are sustainable which means you're less likely to be tempted to give up.

This lack of patience is one of the biggest mental roadblocks to successfully losing weight. People get impatient, they aren't losing weight fast enough for their liking, they blame their diet for not working, and they throw in the towel without giving the diet enough time to prove itself. Change your diet to change your life by having the patience to allow yourself to follow this 27-day plan.

▷ **Stay Positive**

Part of the overweight mentality is only seeing yourself as you are now and wishing you were thinner. Stop wishing and start visualizing. Take time to imagine what you want to look and feel like in 27 days, six months, and even a year down the line. Paint a vivid picture of yourself and your life to let it sink in. Think about how you will feel having lost the weight you want to lose. Is there anything you can't do now that you would do when you've shed those extra pounds? Think about how great that would feel. Use positive visualization to keep a positive outlook on your weight loss journey and yourself.

Another way to use positivity is to surround yourself with it. Have you ever noticed how spending time around a negative ninny who has nothing good to say and only mopes and complains naturally drags your mood down, too? What you surround yourself with is going to influence how you feel. Go to social media, blogs, websites, even website mailing lists, online forums, and support groups; create a Pinterest board; or do anything else you can to surround yourself with positivity. Find influences that focus on positive health and weight loss—not mental self-flagellation for being overweight. Walk past those gossip magazines criticizing celebrities for their supposed body imperfections. Avoid any form of negative body image influences and surround yourself with positive imagery, words, friends, and even videos that align with what you want to achieve.

▷ **Change Your Habits**

Think about your life and your diet. Are there any habits you currently have that are holding you back from losing weight or becoming more active? Habits don't just mean physical actions. Habits can also mean habitual thoughts. A prime example is believing you can't do it or that you'll be overweight for the rest of your life. That one ties in with patience as well. When you don't have the patience to lose weight at a healthy and sustainable rate, you are more likely to feel bad about yourself and think that you can't do it, or it won't happen.

Identify any bad habits or negative habitual thoughts you may have that are holding you back from weight loss success. If you find you have negative thoughts about your weight loss efforts or about yourself, stop the train. Identify the thought; address it by looking at any evidence supporting that thought. Think about whether your friends and loved ones would say the same thing. Chances are there isn't much evidence to back up those thoughts, and your nearest and dearest wouldn't say the same things.

Challenge that thought by replacing it with a positive, motivating thought that will keep you on track.

In addition to bad physical habits and negative
thinking styles, pay attention to your food cravings. It can become such a habit to just give in to
food cravings that you don't even think about it
and just act on impulse. Food cravings aren't all
bad. Sometimes, your body is trying to tell you
something when you do something by making you
crave a certain type of food. For example, if you
have a serious craving for salt or salty food, it
could mean you have an electrolyte imbalance if
you're not drinking enough water and you're
getting dehydrated. However, we also crave things
under certain conditions such as stress. Pay attention to your food cravings and try to figure out
whether you are craving because you are bored,
stressed, unhappy, or whether your craving has a
potentially legitimate reason. If you are craving for
a mental or emotional reason, try to find other
ways to keep busy, give yourself a pick-me-up, or
manage stress.

▷ **Ditch the Overweight Mindset**

What is meant by the "overweight mindset"?
Thinking of yourself as overweight and focusing on

your dissatisfaction with your body has two profound effects on weight loss:

1. When you get those negative feelings about yourself and beat yourself up because you're unhappy with the way you look, your adrenal glands release cortisol. Cortisol is the stress hormone, and it's not doing your waistline any favors. It makes your body store more fat in your midsection (think back to that dangerous abdominal fat we discussed earlier) as opposed to elsewhere.

2. When you focus on how dissatisfied you are with your body and slam yourself for being overweight, you are increasing your avoidance of a healthy diet and exercise. You might even be increasing your chances of gaining weight in the future as well.

The second effect is a biggie. How you think and feel about yourself—your core beliefs—influence how you act. If you feel like you're overweight, have poor self-esteem, and focus on how much you dislike exercise, you're going to be less likely to take action and make the change you truly want to see in your life.

It's important to change the way you view yourself. You need to get into the mindset of adopting a healthy diet and lifestyle because you love and care about your body—not because you loathe it.

▷ **Find Your Why**

This might seem like a no-brainer. You must explore your reasons for wanting to lose weight. The why behind the change is going to be your biggest motivating factor. Try brainstorming to discover all the reasons for your decision to adopt a healthy diet. You can even give each reason a rating from 1–10 to determine how powerful that motivation is. Some people don't mind gaining some weight as they get older, but you're reading this book because you want to make changes to lose the weight. Changing bad habits and creating new ones is hard work. If you're not properly motivated to make them, those changes aren't likely to stick in the long run.

▷ **Use Quality Resources**

This is another big must-do. Yes, you're reading my book to educate yourself about perimenopause and how to lose the dreaded middle-aged spread. However, it's natural to be curious and want to get as much information from as many different sources as you can. That's great! Power to you for wanting to make sure you are healthily changing your diet.

There are so many sources of menopause information out there from magazine articles; blog posts; diet and lifestyle websites; and, of course, dedicated books. You can also consult your physician, a dietitian, or an endocrinologist (specializing in the endocrine system or hormones). With so many sources of information, it can be tempting to hop on the Internet, do a quick web search, and just take the advice from the first few websites that pop up as the gospel truth. However, please don't do that. Not everything you read on the Internet is correct. Not everyone offering advice knows what they are talking about or has any menopause experience to speak from.

At the beginning of this chapter, I urged you to go see your doctor before making any lifestyle or diet changes that would affect your health. Now, I am urging you to be a curious cat—look up information, and equip yourself as well as you can with all the knowledge you need to navigate your way through the various stages of menopause. I am here to help you by offering you knowledge gathered from personal experience and hours of research from quality sources and research studies. Please make sure that any resources you use offer quality information and are trusted sources that won't lead you astray with misinformation, myths, fads, or gimmicks. Your health and happiness truly are worth the time it takes to consult sound resources.

▷ Eat Mindfully

Mindful eating tunes you in with the experience of eating. The idea is to focus on what you are eating and remain in the present while you eat instead of spacing out or focusing on TV or something else that takes your mind off what and how much you're eating. When you're distracted while you're eating, you aren't paying attention to the fact that you're eating at all. This can easily lead to missing your body's cue to tell you you're full, and you may end up overeating before you realize what's happening.

Mindful eating keeps you present and focused on your meal. You don't have to obsessively focus on your plate, but you bring your attention to having the meal. You make the act of eating an experience by noticing and enjoying how tasty the food looks, how delicious it smells, how it tickles your taste buds, and what the food's texture feels like. You are also encouraged to take your time, chew slowly, and enjoy your meal instead of rushing through it at speed, so you can shoot off to take care of other responsibilities.

Another plus of mindful eating is that it brings your attention to what you are choosing to eat and why you're eating. You can't ignore the fact that you're giving in to boredom or stress cravings when you have to sit down and pay attention to the snack or meal. Mindful eating can help you identify your eating habits and the emotions you have toward different types of foods, so you can gain a better understanding of your relationship with food.

▷ **Breathe**

You may be wondering what breathing has to do with dealing with perimenopause and weight loss. The answer: everything.

When your hormones are all muddled up and you're stressed, life can get pretty overwhelming. When you're trying to lose weight and unhelpful habits, thoughts, and a lack of motivation set in, sticking to your plan can seem like an impossible mission. Whenever you feel overwhelmed, stressed, disappointed, or are having a hard time for any reason at all, take a moment to breathe. It is a surprisingly effective way to calm your mind and refocus on the present and your goals.

Belly Breathing Exercise:

- Sit upright or lie on your back, whichever suits you at that moment—as long as you're comfortable.
- Place one hand on your belly and then the other hand on your chest.
- As you breathe in and out, focus on drawing your breath into your belly instead of your chest.
- Breathe in through your nose for approximately four seconds.
- Hold your breath for two seconds.
- Breathe out for six seconds.
- As you breathe in and out, the hand on your belly should rise and fall while the hand on your chest should stay relatively still.

Don't wait until everything is just right. It will never be perfect. There will always be challenges, obstacles, and less-than-perfect conditions. So what. Get started now.

— M.V. HANSEN

4

PREPARING FOR A HEALTHY DIET: DAY 2

Preparing yourself for perimenopause, or helping you deal with it if you're already in its grip, is to know what your symptoms are and keeping track of them. Knowing what your symptoms are is all good and well, but you won't necessarily know if they are getting worse unless you are tracking them.

Use the template below to identify your perimenopause symptoms and track them. When you have an idea of what your symptoms are and what their severity is, you can consult your physician or a specialist for advice on how to best treat them and any possible underlying causes.

Important Note: You may be having symptoms you identify as being caused by perimenopause, but this time of hormonal change may not be the actual cause. Discussing your symptoms with a doctor can help rule out any other possible causes.

PERIMENOPAUSE SYMPTOM TRACKER

You can use a daily diary or planner to track your symptoms by printing the table below and attaching it to a new page for each new day. You can also design and print out a chart to use for tracking your symptoms for a whole month. That approach allows you to see the bigger picture at a glance but won't record the finer details of the checker below. If you do decide to create a printable chart on an A4 page in landscape orientation, create 30 or 31 columns under a "day of the month" section and note only the severity of the symptom in general for the whole day.

Symptom scoring guideline:

Rate your symptoms with a value of 0 to 10, with 10 being greatly affected, 0 being not at all affected, 5 being moderately affected.

Assign one of the scores above to each symptom you experience on any particular day and fill in the symptom checker every single day. Doing this will give you greater insight as to which symptoms you are experiencing, their frequency, and their severity.

Using the specific checker below, fill the frequency by noting how many times during the day you felt that symptom and the duration by noting how long the symptom lasted. Some symptoms won't have a frequency or duration, such as loss of or thinning of hair. In those instances, you can make a note if you notice these changes have occurred and just jot it down if you think it's getting worse.

Day of the Month:_____

Symptom	Severity	Frequency	Duration
Menstrual Cycle Symptoms			
Only spotting during your period			
Light period			
Medium period			
Heavy period			
Breakthrough bleeding between periods			

Physical Symptoms			
Abdominal or pelvic pain			
Ache or pimples			
An increase in whiskery hair on your chin and jawline			
Backache			
Bloating (similar to PMS bloating)			
Breasts that are swollen or tender/painful			
Dry skin or skin that feels papery			
Fatigue or a lack of energy			
Food cravings or overeating (It may be interesting to jot down the specific foods you are craving on any given day.)			
Heart palpitations (feeling as if your heart is beating faster, fluttering, or pounding)			

Hot flashes (at night)			
Hot flashes (during the daytime)			
Insomnia (unable to fall asleep, stay asleep, or go back to sleep after waking up in the early hours)			
Loss of or lowered sex drive/desire			
Loss of or thinning of your hair			
Migraines or headaches (Circle the one you are experiencing.)			
Muscle and/or joint stiffness or pain			
Nausea			
Night sweats			
Pain during sex			
Problems with bladder control			
Sleep disturbances (waking up frequently during the night)			
Vaginal discharge			
Vaginal dryness			
Weight gain			
Your voice is getting deeper.			

Emotional and Mental Symptoms			
Anxiousness			
Brain fog or difficulties concentrating			
Emotional outbursts			
Feeling stressed or overwhelmed			
Feeling tearful or crying			
Feeling depressed or sad			
Getting angry quickly or having a short temper			
Grumpiness/irritability			
Having relationship troubles			
Memory problems/loss			
Mood swings			
Withdrawing/being antisocial			

Digital Symptom Trackers

With technology continually progressing, you can take advantage of symptom tracker applications that are downloadable straight to your smartphone. This puts perimenopause symptom tracking at your fingertips at any point in the day. You can search for symptom trackers on the App Store or Google Play. Keep in mind to pick a tracking app that suits your needs—whether you want something simple or that offers more features, whether you want a paid app, or something free to use. To make the experience easier and get exactly what you want from it, do a little research, read reviews, and check out features for different apps before deciding.

Rule One is never quit. Rule Two is: refer to Rule One. Cake happens, but as long as you remember those rules, you'll be OK.

— UNKNOWN

5

PREPARING FOR A HEALTHY DIET: DAY 3

In this chapter, I'm going to cover calorie counting and the benefits of recording and watching your calories. Many people find keeping track of their calories helpful to help them control their weight in the long run. That's not to say you have to become a compulsive calorie counter and stick to a limit down to the last calorie. It's just a helpful way to make sure you don't end up eating too many calories. This might seem like a hard and unnecessary thing at first, however, if I told you weight loss is a very simple science of calories in vs. calories out, would you believe me? Yes, you have heard that one before, I know. We will focus heavily on the quality and source of our calories later which is the bit that really matters.

We've already established that to lose weight, you need to create a modest calorie deficit. Recording what you eat and how many calories you're eating can help you make better food choices and control portion sizes. We have to begin by understanding what your regular daily food choices are and how many calories you're eating on average. You might just be surprised at how many calories some types of food contains and that you might be eating more than you think.

Calorie counting is not meant to be a food-shaming exercise. What you're trying to do is figure out what your eating habits are right now. It's easier to change habits when you understand where changes need to be made, and you can only do that by finding out what you're eating and where your calories are coming from. I cannot stress enough that you should do this exercise from a judgment-free zone.

It can be an eye-opener to track your choices and calories in a food diary. Some women are drawn into feelings of guilt and shame when they realize what and how much they are eating. That is not what the intention here is at all. You are simply observing as if looking in from the outside. Your food choices don't define who you are, and they can be changed, so be open and honest with yourself without falling into the trap of judging yourself for the choices you're making right now. Focus on your goal of learning to make healthier choices going forward.

HOW CALORIE TRACKING IS HELPFUL

Counting calories has gained a bit of a bad reputation. When you think about counting calories, you probably immediately think of typical diets of micro portions and food that isn't tantalizing to your taste buds. It's also linked to crash diets and extreme restrictions. On top of the less-than-stellar reputation calorie tracking has, there are so many diets out there that focus on specific food groups being restricted or even cut out. An example is the keto diet which vilifies carbohydrates. These food group restrictive diets encourage people to develop unhealthy relationships by labeling foods as "good" or "bad." In reality, food isn't good or bad unless it contains potentially harmful ingredients. Food is fuel for your body—that's it.

Sure, the quality of the fuel you choose to put into your body affects your health, but it's not necessarily going to affect your weight and body fat. The part of food, nutritious or not, that affects your weight is the calorie content, and that's why counting calories can be so useful. Before we dive into why counting calories can be good for losing weight and maintaining healthy weight results once you reach your goal, let's get a better understanding of calories.

What Are Calories?

A calorie is a unit used to measure the energy we get from the food we eat. Everything you eat and drink, except for water, counts toward your daily calorie intake. That morning cup of coffee? Yes, that teaspoon of coffee and splash of milk comes with a small calorie price. Most foods measure their energy value in kilocalories or Kcal, even though we usually just refer to them as calories and leave the kilo part off.

I mentioned earlier that food is neither good nor bad —there is just quality. Not all calories are created equal, and that is where the quality part comes in. When it comes to weight management, a calorie will be a calorie no matter whether it comes from a slice of cake or a salad.

If a calorie is a calorie whether it comes from sugar-coated cereal or oatmeal, why does the quality matter in terms of weight loss? This comes down to a matter of quality versus quantity. The quality of the calories you eat has a hand to play in how much you eat. Wait, what? Can't you just eat the same number of calories irrespective of where they come from? Yes, you can, but let me explain why it doesn't work that way.

Remember I mentioned malnutrition in Chapter 2 when I was discussing why a calorie deficit that's too big is harmful to your health? The same goes for the quality of the calories you fuel your body with. For instance, a slice of white bread made from refined flour doesn't have the same nutritional value as a slice of whole grain bread even if the calorie value is relatively similar.

The nutrients and fiber in the food you eat affect your hormones, metabolism, and hunger. Nutrient-dense foods are likely to leave you feeling more satisfied for longer after a meal. On the other hand, a meal of food offering empty calories and little fiber or nutrition is likely to give you a blood sugar spike/crash and make you feel hungry sooner, leaving you feeling less healthy overall because your body is not getting the nutrition it needs.

When you're counting calories, the quality of your calories makes all the difference to your success. Nobody likes feeling hungry, and that makes it harder to create and maintain a calorie deficit for weight loss. When you fill yourself up on empty calories, added sugar, and refined carbohydrates offering little fiber, you're going to feel hungry and want to eat more instead of sticking to your calorie limit.

Now that we've established what calories are and why quality is so important, let's begin with what the benefits of counting calories are.

Counting Calories: The Benefits

▷ **Your Daily Caloric Needs**

To be able to count calories effectively for weight loss, you need to know how many you need per day. Just counting the number of calories in the food you eat isn't going to do much if you don't know where you should cap it off for the day.

▷ **You Learn the Caloric Difference**

Counting calories is a great way to open your eyes to how many calories different types of food contain. Many people may look at a small portion of "junk food," such as a small packet of potato chips, and not be bothered by the number of calories they think they're consuming. Why? Well, it's a small portion, right? How can a small amount of food contain all that many calories? This is one of the biggest and generally most common mistakes people make when trying to judge what they can or can't eat. A good example is a 1.5-ounce packet of potato chips averages around 240 calories. 1.5 ounces of fresh apple, on the other hand, offers only 22.5 calories, but it packs a much bigger nutritional punch.

▷ **Better Choices Come Easier**

Along with learning that not all foods are created equal and that you pay a hefty calorie price for surprisingly small portions of some foods, you also learn to make better choices. When you start counting calories, you take note of what kinds of foods are calorie-heavy and which aren't. You learn what you can eat more of and what you can only get away with a small amount of. You learn to budget your calories if you know you are going to be indulging in high-calorie foods: "I'm having cheese-cake for dessert after dinner, so I'm not going to have ice cream after lunch."

I'm not here to encourage going hungry to lose weight. By following a healthy diet, you can eat without feeling guilty or ending up "hangry." Counting calories teaches you to make better food choices by choosing nutrient-dense, healthy, and filling foods that won't break the calorie bank and help you reach your weight loss goal.

▷ **You Downsize Your Portions**

Let's face it: You're not always going to make healthy food choices. We all enjoy fast food, snacks, and treats from time to time, but what about those weight loss plans? Won't indulging a little bit now and then sabotage what you're trying to achieve? Not at all. That is what calorie counting will help you with.

When you can't, or don't want to, necessarily opt for the healthiest item on the menu, counting calories helps you keep portion sizes in perspective. Have you ever noticed how large some fast food or restaurant portions are? Counting calories allows you to divide that big portion into smaller, waistline-friendly portions and you can just take the rest home and enjoy it as part of your calorie budget tomorrow.

TRACKING YOUR FOOD

Tracking your calories and the food you eat go hand in hand with each other. How can you track your calories if you aren't tracking the food you're eating? This is where keeping a food journal comes in handy, and part of your preparation for taking control of your diet by making changes is to know what your current diet is like.

Let's talk seriously about food journaling for a moment. It's important to begin recording what you are eating and how many calories you're consuming before you adopt a new, healthy diet. This step will help you establish a baseline and give you a better understanding of where your diet needs to be tweaked. This exercise isn't meant to food-shame your current choices, and it's not meant to make you feel guilty.

Remember what I said earlier? Food isn't good or bad: It's simply fuel for your body. There is high-quality and poor-quality fuel, but that doesn't make the food itself good or bad. Labeling food as good and bad creates a distorted relationship with food, and that's not going to help get you anywhere. It can, in fact, lead to obsessive or disordered eating habits, and that's definitely not what I want for you. What we're trying to do is improve the quality of your choices for the majority of the time while allowing you to indulge now and then so that you don't feel deprived.

Food Journaling Exercise

- Grab a journal and jot down every single thing you eat and drink throughout the day. You should ideally do this every day for about a week.
- Note down when you are eating what and, if you can determine the reason, why you are eating it. This step can help you identify times of day you may be more hungry or susceptible to giving in to cravings. It could also help you figure out if you are reaching for a snack because of mental or emotional reasons, such as stress.
- It may be tempting to change your eating habits during this time because your attention is suddenly drawn to your eating habits, plus, you may be surprised at what you're eating and how many calories you're taking in. Resist that temptation.
- Be completely honest with yourself. Don't

skip anything—not even if you just take a
bite of someone else's food.

Important Note: Going forward, even after you
have recorded a week of eating in your food journal
to establish a baseline, keep recording what you eat
and drink. If you don't do this all the time, that's
okay. Even tracking your eating habits sporadically
can help keep you on track and improve your weight
loss and weight maintenance.

If keeping a physical food journal isn't your thing, go
digital. Technology is a wondrous thing. It can help
make almost every part of your life easier and more
convenient. There are a variety of food tracking
websites and even mobile apps that allow you to
easily record food, beverages, amounts, and calories
all at the same time. Some will even give you a
breakdown of your macronutrient split. Macros
refer to fat, protein, and carbohydrates: The three
nutrients your body needs in larger amounts every
day. You may even be able to see your micronutrients, or vitamins and minerals, so you can keep track
of whether you are getting enough of those in to
support optimum health.

Tracking Portions

Recording your daily calorie intake means tracking your portion sizes. Portions and servings often get mixed up because not everybody knows the difference. It's worth knowing the difference between the two so I'll explain it quickly:

- A portion is how much you choose to eat.
- A serving is how much food a manufacturer lists under their nutritional information label on the package.

The serving size on labels is based on the recommended daily allowance (RDA), also known as the recommended daily intake (RDI), which is set by the Food and Nutrition Board of the Institute of Medicine. RDA refers to the recommended calories, macronutrients, and micronutrients an adult needs per day to stay healthy. If you look at the nutritional label for a food item, the table will list the calories and nutrition with a corresponding percentage. That percentage is the percentage of what you should be getting daily.

Interestingly, portion sizes have gradually increased over the last few decades, leading to adults eating more calories per day than they need. Consider my earlier comment on large restaurant portions. Many people will clean their plates even though the portion size is way bigger than it should be.

That being said, it can be difficult to estimate what a portion size of a specific food should look like—especially with processed foods being so abundant and filled with empty calories. Counting calories can help you determine what your portion size should be based on the number of calories in a portion of a particular food and how many calories you should be eating.

Keeping track of your portions will mean measuring the amount of food you're eating. How do you go about it (considering eye-balling doesn't count)?

- Measuring cups and spoons
- Kitchen scales
- Comparisons

When talking about comparisons, you are comparing the amount of a specific food you are eating to a common household item as a way of judging the nutrition by sight. This isn't as accurate as using scales or measuring cups, but it will work in a pinch. Here are some common comparisons:

One Serving Of:	Size comparison item:
Vegetables—about ½ a cup	A standard computer mouse
Leafy green vegetables—about 1 cup	A baseball
Fresh fruit—about ½ a cup	A tennis ball
Fish—3 ounces	A checkbook
Meat—3 ounces	A deck of cards
Cheese—1.5 ounces	A tube of lipstick
Pasta or rice—½ a cup	A rounded handful or a standard computer mouse
Olive oil—1 teaspoon	Your fingertip
Peanut butter—2 tablespoons	A ping pong ball

Commit to the process no matter how long it takes, and the payoffs and benefits can be greater than anything you have ever imagined.

— LIZ JOSEFSBERG

6

PREPARING FOR A HEALTHY DIET: DAY 4

In the previous preparation chapters, we covered how to get into a healthy diet mindset, track your perimenopause symptoms, and track your food and calories. In this chapter, I'm going to take you through how to calculate your daily caloric needs and measure your body from the start of your weight loss journey and periodically throughout to measure your progress.

Why can't you just use your trusty bathroom scale to measure your weight loss progress? Let me tell you something: That bathroom scale isn't as trusty as you might think it is. I'm not saying it will present you with an incorrect number, but it will tell you white lies about your weight loss. You might be asking, "How can a piece of equipment like a scale lie?" It's not a conscious being, so it can't think for itself and decide to tell you something that isn't true.

Yes, a scale can't think for itself and tell you a lie in the most basic sense of the word, but it can still deceive you when you step on it. You see, muscle is denser than fat, and therefore, it weighs more. If you go into your kitchen and compare a pound of butter with a pound of fillet steak, which is smaller? The steak, of course.

Exercise is a vital part of holistic health, and you should be getting regular exercise according to the CDC's recommended guidelines we discussed earlier. When you get fitter and build muscle, it will add to your weight while losing fat will reduce your weight. Essentially, as you gain muscle at the same time as you lose fat, your scale may tell you that you haven't lost much at all. Meanwhile, back at the ranch, you are losing more body fat than it's telling you because it's not just telling you how much fat you're losing. Scales don't discriminate—they don't take your intentions into account and tell you what you really want to know. This can make it seem like you're not losing body fat as quickly as you actually are. In fact, the number may not seem to budge at times. That doesn't necessarily mean you're not losing weight; it just means you're gaining muscle while losing fat, and the two are canceling each other out.

Measuring your progress is vitally important for your weight loss success. The biggest motivator to keep us working toward our goals is when we can see we're getting there. Using your bathroom scale alone won't be a hugely motivating factor, and you need to find ways to more accurately gauge how much body fat you're losing. I'm going to tell you how to do just that.

PHYSICAL MEASUREMENTS

One of the most accurate ways of measuring your weight loss progress is to take physical measurements of your body. The scale may not tell you that your waist is getting smaller, but a measuring tape will. As you lose body fat, both abdominal and the subcutaneous layer of fat under your skin, your measurements will gradually shrink. What about the increase in muscle size as you build muscle from following a regular exercise regimen? Muscle doesn't take up nearly as much space as fat, pound for pound, and building muscle doesn't happen overnight. You aren't going to start lunges and squats today and have enormous bodybuilder legs by next week. Muscle growth is a slow process, and you're not likely to build enough muscle to combat body fat shrinkage. You'll still see noticeable results even if you're building muscle at the same time as losing body fat.

It's a good idea to track your progress by jotting down your measurements, so you can refer back to the previous measurements to see how they stack up. It's not a good idea, however, to become addicted to that measuring tape and measure yourself every day. Just like weighing yourself daily can be an incredibly distressing and disheartening exercise, measuring yourself every day could leave your motivation in shreds.

Your body changes every single day because of factors like bloating and water retention. This is especially true while you're going through perimenopause, and your hormones are fluctuating. Hormones can make you retain more water today than you did yesterday and can cause digestive issues which lead to bloating. Water retention not only makes you appear heavier on the scale—it causes your body's cells, including fat cells, to swell up. This can make your body measurements—especially around the hips, thighs, and tummy—seem to creep up when you aren't gaining fat.

How often you measure yourself is entirely up to you as long as it's no more than once per week. If you're going to measure yourself weekly, make sure it's on the same day of the week and at the same time of day every single time. Why does the time of day matter? Your body doesn't only change each day: It undergoes changes during the day. After a night's sleep, your body has lost a lot of water through breathing because you exhale tiny droplets of water vapor every time you breathe out. By the time you have woken up in the morning, you will weigh less than you did the night before because of that water loss. You are also less bloated because it's been several hours since your last meal, and your digestive system has had time to process everything and calm down again. As a rule of thumb, you should weigh and measure yourself first thing in the morning after you have gotten up and gone to the bathroom but before you drink or eat anything.

Important Notes:

- It's so important to make sure you take your initial weight, measurements, and pictures of yourself before you start your weight loss journey. These create a baseline for you to track your progress, and you can look back at your first measurements to see how far you have come and how much your body has changed.

- When measuring your body with a measuring tape, ensure the tape is snug but not pulled too tightly. The tape should not be pressing into your skin—just lightly against it.

Chest/Bust: Wrap the measuring tape around your chest, keeping it in line with your nipple. Take your chest measurement at the side of your ribs (under your arm).

Waist: Measure the smallest part of your waist, usually half an inch above your belly button. Make sure the tape is level all the way around. You should take the measurement by feel, as trying to look down could bunch your midsection up and give you a false measurement.

Important Note: Your waist is the part of your body that will produce the least accurate measurement of progress. Many women look to their midsection for progress because it's the part we generally want to slim down the most. However, your waist measurements could be misleading because of bloating which results from eating or from your menstrual cycle—whether you're PMS or actively menstruating. Hormonal fluctuations during perimenopause could cause bloating outside of your period as well, so don't use your waist measurement as a conclusive summary of your weight loss progress.

Hips: Measure your hips at the widest part. Keep the measuring tape level all the way around.

Thighs: You should measure only one thigh because if one gets slimmer, the other one is doing the same. Measure at the widest part of your thigh, near the top, and make sure the tape is level all the way around.

Arms: Measure about six inches (15 cm) up your arm from the tip of your elbow. This should take you to roughly the middle of your upper arm. Make sure the tape remains level.

Important Note: When measuring your arms and thighs, it's important to measure the same arm and thigh every time. The human body is a wondrous thing, and one side of your body is bigger than the other. It's not noticeable to the naked eye, but a measuring tape might show you the difference.

VISUAL MEASUREMENTS

Seeing the numbers on the scale and the measuring tape come down is always a great feeling, but human beings are visual creatures. We want to see the progress we are making—not just according to numbers. This is why visual measurements can be so impactful and motivating. There are two ways to visually keep track of your progress:

Take Pictures: You must have seen before-and-after weight loss photos of people posting their weight loss success stories online. You can do the same as a visual record of your weight loss. Don't worry: You don't have to post your pictures online. You can keep them private because they're for your personal use. You should take pictures of yourself from different angles such as from the front, back (if you can), and sides. It's useful to ask a friend to help you, but you can also use a full-length mirror. You can take photos in your underwear or tight-fitting clothing to give you an accurate visual. Don't take the photos wearing loose or baggy clothing because you won't be able to see the slimming down happening.

Clothing Sizes: If taking photos isn't really your thing, why not look at your clothing to measure your progress? There is nothing that proves you are losing body fat other than the fit of your clothes. You can pick an outfit that isn't particularly comfortable or could be a little too small at the moment. Put it on and take note of how it fits. A month down the line, put that same outfit on again and see how it fits now. As you lose weight, you should notice waistbands fitting better and shirts getting looser.

WORKING OUT YOUR DAILY CALORIC NEEDS

We've discussed counting calories and working with a calorie deficit, but before you can start working with a calorie budget and create a deficit, you need to know what your daily caloric needs are. There are two different parts to working out what your daily calories should be. First, you have to work out your basal metabolic rate, and then, you use that result and your physical activity level to get to an overall total. These formulas are easy to use and will give you an idea of what you should be eating.

Important Note: These formulas are by no means 100% accurate. They have been created and tweaked over time to be used as a guideline that is as accurate as it can be without specialized medical testing. The answers will give you a good starting point to begin changing your diet to lose weight. You can always make gradual changes to how many calories you eat if you find you aren't getting the results you want. Interestingly, if you have ever been on a FAD diet, this is the formula that would be used to work out calorie reduction. Unfortunately, what you probably do not know is that after you achieve your desired weight you need to adjust your calories up to your normal requirements in order to maintain the weight forever. With this tool you will be able to work out exactly how many calories you can allow yourself to have, how to manage your portions and how to be able to have an occasional treat without feeling guilty.

Basal Metabolic Rate

Your basal metabolic rate, also called your BMR, is the bare minimum of calories you need to perform life-sustaining bodily functions to remain healthy. It doesn't take into account any additional calories you burn through physical activity. These life-sustaining functions include, but are not limited to, involuntary internal goings-on like metabolizing food, breathing, keeping your heart beating to pump blood, and brain function. Basal metabolic rate doesn't calculate any physical activity. It's calculated based purely on your body at rest.

There have been several BMR formulas developed over time—the first of which is called the Harris-Benedict equation. The formula considered the most accurate is the Mifflin-St. Jeor equation. This is the third revision of the Harris-Benedict equation. You can easily look up BMR calculators online, but let's use the Mifflin-St. Jeor equation to demonstrate how your BMR is calculated. This equation is generally accurate to within 10% of the result you would get using a medical device.

Did You Know?: BMR calculation formulas differ slightly between men and women. This is due to the difference in body composition, as men tend to have more muscle while women tend to have more body fat. It may be frustrating that women carry more body fat than men. What do you have to thank for this? Evolution. Women have evolved to carry more body fat to ensure their survival during harsh times. Even though our lifestyle has evolved to need and also covet less body fat, evolution hasn't grasped that yet.

Mifflin-St. Jeor equation for women:

(15.88 × height in inches) + (4.536 × weight in lbs) − (5 × age) − 161

or in metric values

(10 x weight in kgs) + (6.25 x height in cms) - (5 x age) - 161

If a 45-year-old woman stands 5 foot, 7 inches tall and weighs 180 pounds, her BMR would be calculated as:

- (15.88 x 79 inches) + (4.536 x 180 pounds) - (5 x 45) - 161
- 1,254.52 + 816.48 - 225 - 161 = a BMR of 1,685 calories per day

Using the above example, work out your own BMR.

Total Daily Energy Expenditure (TDEE)

Now that you can work out your BMR, let's move on to calculating your overall calorie requirements for the day, also called total daily energy expenditure or TDEE. This is calculated by multiplying your BMR by a number based on your average daily activity level.

- Do you lead a sedentary lifestyle where you don't get much physical activity if any? - BMR x 1.2
- Do you get light physical activity 1–3 days per week? - BMR x 1.375
- Do you get moderate-intensity exercise 3–5 days per week? - BMR x 1.55
- Do you get vigorous-intensity exercise 6–7 days per week? - BMR x 1.725
- Do you get vigorous-intensity exercise 6–7 days per week and work a physically demanding job or exercise at a vigorous intensity twice per day? - BMR x 1.9

Let's go back to the previous example of the same woman used in the BMR calculation. Let's say she leads a sedentary lifestyle.

BMR 1,685 x 1.2 = 2,022 total daily calorie expenditure: This is the number of calories she needs to eat per day to maintain that weight.

As a conservative calculation, unless you are a professional athlete, use the light activity number as your guidance.

Using the above example, work out your own TDEE.

Online TDEE calculators will help if you need a little shortcut to establish how many calories you need.

Calculating a Calorie Deficit

As I touched on in Chapter 1, to lose weight, you need to consume fewer calories than you'll need for maintaining your current weight. This requires a calorie deficit. I warned of the dangers of eating too few calories, so how much is enough to safely lose weight and stay healthy?

A good rule of thumb is to cut your calories by 15–20% per day to lose a gradual and healthy amount of weight per week. If you want to lose more body fat per week, you will need to cut your calories a little more, but 15–20% should do the trick for healthy weight loss.

Rest assured, based on these conservative numbers and 20% calorie deficit, you will see results quickly. The meal plan I've provided you in Chapter 8 is calculated to this level, but it's only a guideline. It's meant to help you figure out your own calorie needs and work with your diet accordingly.

Important Note: I cannot reiterate this enough throughout this book. Each woman's body is different and will have a different metabolic rate. These formulas and deficit guidelines are generalized and only meant to give you an idea of how to manage your weight loss. If you find you aren't losing up to two pounds per week by cutting your daily calories by 15–20%, try cutting them down further but only in small increments until you achieve your result. Take it easy and listen to your body and how you feel. Keep in mind that the emphasis here is on healthy weight loss which happens gradually. I know it's tempting to want to lose weight faster. Losing weight too fast can be detrimental to your health and could cause you to gain weight again when you increase your calorie intake once you have lost the weight you want to lose. Gradual weight loss will also make it easier to keep the pounds off once you bring your calories back up to a maintenance level.

It is never too late to be what you might have been.

— GEORGE ELLIOT

7

PREPARING FOR A HEALTHY DIET: DAY 5

In this chapter, I will take you through the fifth and final phase of preparing to adopt a new, healthy diet. You've done a great job preparing yourself mentally and discovering how to calculate your caloric needs for weight loss. Now, it's time to set some weight loss, and even fitness, goals. For this, we'll use the principle of SMART goals.

SETTING SMART GOALS

The SMART goals principle is used to help you set goals properly. Have you ever wondered why giving up New Year's resolutions has become such a cliché and why it's so hard, if not impossible, to stick to them? More often than not, it's because the goals being set are not SMART. They are not set properly according to certain criteria that make it easier to stay motivated and achieve them. I really want you to achieve your goal of losing weight and keeping it off during perimenopause—and for the rest of your life— so I'm going to walk you through setting effective SMART goals.

There are five pillars to the SMART goal principle:

- Specific
- Measurable
- Attainable
- Realistic
- Time-Bound

Let's break it down further to understand what each pillar means exactly, and why you should be setting your goals this way.

Specific

Many people fail to specify their goals properly which leads them to fail at achieving them. Vague goals don't tell you exactly where you're going: They just give you a general idea. Think of your weight loss journey as a road trip. Let's say you are in Jacksonville, Florida, and you want to go to San Francisco, California. Many people set a goal of going to California. However, how are they going to get to San Francisco if they don't define exactly where they are going? The same goes for weight loss. Many people set themselves the goal of "weight loss," but they don't specify how much weight they want to lose. When you set your weight loss goal, define your goal in terms of how much weight you want to lose or how many dress sizes you'd want to go down. This gives you an ultimately clear vision of what you are working toward.

Measurable

This part ties in with setting specific goals. You need to measure your progress toward your goal to see how far you have come and how far you still have to go. When you just say you want to "lose weight," you can measure your weight loss in terms of you have lost five pounds or gone down half a dress size or a dress size. However, if you don't have a clear vision of what your goal is, what does losing five pounds mean or going down half a dress size mean? How much progress have you made toward reaching your goal, and how far do you still have to go before you get there?

Another consideration for measurable goals is deciding how you are going to measure your progress. Are you going to measure your weight loss in pounds, dress size, or body measurements? You should pick a form of measurement and stick to it throughout your weight loss to keep a consistent measure of your progress.

Attainable

Do you have the means and ability to reach your goal? By means, I am referring to the resources, time, and also motivation needed to reach a goal. For weight loss, resources may not be relevant, but time and motivation are. If you aren't sufficiently motivated to lose weight, you aren't likely to put in the effort required to achieve weight loss. If you are incorporating exercise into your weight loss plan, do you have the time to get the recommended amount of exercise per week?

Realistic

So many people fall short when it comes to setting realistic goals. Let's use the same example used in the previous chapter of the 45-year-old woman who is 5 foot 7 inches tall and weighs 180 pounds. Let's also say she has a medium frame. She wants to lose 70 pounds to reach her goal weight of 110 pounds and become petite like a celebrity she admires. She has the motivation to stick to a diet and exercise plan; the time to fit exercise into her daily schedule; and the time to prepare fresh, healthy meals. Is losing 70 pounds and being petite a realistic goal for her? The unfortunate truth is that it isn't. Losing 70 pounds would put her at a BMI of 17.2 which is classified as underweight. Furthermore, with having a medium frame, her ideal of being petite isn't going to happen because you cannot change your bone structure no matter how much weight you lose.

For her to set a realistic goal, she needs to take her current BMI and her physical frame into account. At 180 pounds, her BMI is 28.2, which classifies her as overweight. A realistic goal would be to aim for a weight loss of 25–40 pounds to get into a BMI that is in a healthy range.

Time-Bound

The last pillar of the SMART goals principle is time-bound. For you to reach your goal, you need to set some type of time limit for reaching it. If you don't set a realistic time limit for reaching your goal, you could spend the rest of your life trying to lose the weight you want to lose. Deciding how long you will give yourself to reach your goal amps up your motivation and makes you hold yourself accountable for your actions that lead to success.

Did you notice I said a realistic time limit? Just like your goal needs to be realistic, you need to be realistic about how much time you're going to give yourself to achieve it. Let's once again return to our example woman and say she wants to lose 30 pounds. The hormonal upset of perimenopause can make it harder to lose weight than when you were younger. Weight loss also needs to happen at a safe, gradual rate. Taking those two factors into account, realistically, she should be aiming for a one-pound weight loss per week. Therefore, she should set the time limit for reaching her goal at 30 weeks.

Unfortunately, 30 weeks may seem like a long time, and impatience often gets the better of people. The desire for instant gratification and fast results often leads to setting time limits that aren't realistic and only sets you up for failure. What happens when you don't reach your goal in the time you've set yourself to do it? You become despondent, beat yourself up, and give up because you decide you simply cannot lose the amount of overall weight you want to lose.

ADDITIONAL GOAL-SETTING TIPS

▷ **Set Long-Term Goals**

Use your overall goal of losing the total amount of weight you want to lose and maintaining that weight as your long-term goal. You've given yourself a realistic timeframe in which to achieve that goal, and now, you need to work toward getting there.

▷ **Set Short-Term Goals**

You've set your long-term goal, and now, it's time to break that goal up into smaller achievements to help you get there. Breaking a large, long-term goal up into smaller chunks makes it seem less daunting. You can lose motivation along the way when you are staring this big goal in the face, and you're just toiling away at achieving it. By setting milestones to achieve along the way, you are more likely to stay motivated because it feels good to reach each of those milestones. You can keep your long-term goal in sight, but try to focus on the smaller goals.

▷ Keep Sight of the Bigger Picture

Your primary goal may be weight loss, but you should keep sight of the bigger picture. Losing weight will improve your overall health and reduce your risk of diseases while increasing your longevity. Including exercise will help improve your fitness which also reduces your risk of health problems and will improve your mobility, flexibility, and range of motion. Keeping the bigger picture in sight will further motivate you to keep at it—even when things aren't going smoothly.

▷ Don't Rush

It's better for your health and chances of keeping the weight off if you take things slow. If you've ever tried a crash diet to lose a substantial amount of weight in a short time, you will know how frustrating it is when the weight piles right back on the moment you stop the strict diet. Losing weight gradually could be your key to successfully losing the weight and also keeping it off. Why? You are developing lifelong, healthy habits that aren't going to go out the window once you've reached your goal weight. After all, you don't just want to enjoy your weight loss for a week or two before your weight starts creeping up again. You want to enjoy your weight loss for the rest of your life.

WHAT'S THE NEXT STEP?

You've now gone through the five phases of preparing to adopt a healthy diet and lifestyle. You have done the following:

- You've mentally prepared to change current habits and develop new ones by changing your attitude.
- You've identified and tracked your perimenopause symptoms to find ways to deal with them, so they don't sap your motivation.
- You've tracked your calorie intake, the types of food you eat, and identified when you eat and why you're eating to identify where your diet needs to be tweaked.
- You've calculated your daily caloric needs and the deficit you need to create to lose weight.
- You've set SMART weight loss and health goals to make sure you are setting the right goals and can effectively reach them.

Now, it's time to take on the task of adopting a healthier diet and lifestyle, and I'm going to help you by providing you with a three-week healthy diet meal plan. The foods and meals are delicious, nutritious, and form part of a balanced diet. They are based on a combination of the Mediterranean diet and anti-inflammatory food principles. There is no starving yourself on a severely restrictive diet—only wholesome food that will tantalize your taste buds. Your calories have been split in a balanced way: 40/30/30 ratio. 40% of your calories will come from carbs, 30% from protein, and 30% from fats.

As you may notice the recipes are mainly vegetarian. I found this kind of combination was found to be most helpful for many women in order to get their weight and perimenopausal symptoms under control. I have since adopted a vegan lifestyle, but you absolutely do not have to. As long as you are aware of how many calories you require, and split your calories in a balanced way, you can try designing your own meals. There are a variety of trackers and apps available that will help you become very aware of how big your portions should be, based on your calorie requirements. With time, you will not need to count anything anymore and just by looking at a plate of food you will know how many calories it contains. You will intuitively know how big your portions should be in order to leave you satisfied. Practice these skills, until they become your new habit. This will help you achieve your goals, and reach for new ones.

Please keep in mind that you are doing this for the long haul. You want to achieve lasting results so that you don't end up in an unhealthy cycle of yo-yo dieting. Keep yourself motivated by tracking your progress and evaluate how you feel all the time. How are you doing?

- Are you struggling or is this easy-peasy lemon squeezy?
- Do you need to adjust your short-term goals to break them up into smaller, more manageable milestones?
- Do you need to find some support to keep you accountable for taking the action and making the changes needed to achieve your goal?

Keep tabs on how you feel—physically, mentally, and emotionally. You may need to make some adjustments to your original plan, but that's okay. The important thing is to keep going to reach your goal and not give up.

You can do this. You've got this: Trust me. I believe in you, and you should believe in yourself because your health and happiness are worth it!

Believe and act as if it were impossible to fail.

— CHARLES KETTERING

8

21-DAY MEAL PLAN

MEAL PLAN WEEK 1

Day	Meals
Monday	
Breakfast	Oatmeal with cinnamon and raisins
Lunch	Whole wheat feta and veggie sandwich
Dinner	Vegetable tacos with cilantro sauce
Snack	Blueberry banana smoothie

Tuesday	
Breakfast	Loaded vegetable omelet
Lunch	Vegetable tacos with cilantro sauce
Dinner	Zucchini zoodles with parmesan
Snack	Peanut butter and celery snack

Wednesday	
Breakfast	Avocado toast with poached eggs
Lunch	Zucchini "zoodles" with parmesan
Dinner	Lentil and veggie soup
Snack	Mixed berries and yogurt

Thursday	
Breakfast	Fruit and veggie smoothie
Lunch	Lentil and veggie soup
Dinner	Cauliflower steaks with chimichurri sauce
Snack	Granola and berries bowl

Friday	
Breakfast	Loaded vegetable omelet
Lunch	Cauliflower steaks with chimichurri sauce
Dinner	Vegetarian one-pot chili
Snack	Apple and peanut butter stacks

Saturday	
Breakfast	Fruit and nuts breakfast bowl
Lunch	Vegetarian one-pot chili
Dinner	Quick black bean salad
Snack	Toast with almond butter and banana
Sunday	
Breakfast	Oatmeal with cinnamon and raisins
Lunch	Chickpea and quinoa bowl
Dinner	Thai pumpkin curry
Snack	Carrot sticks and homemade hummus

MEAL PLAN WEEK 2

Day	Meals
Monday	
Breakfast	Loaded vegetable omelet
Lunch	Whole wheat feta and veggie sandwich
Dinner	Vegetarian one-pot- chili
Snack	Blueberry banana smoothie

Tuesday	
Breakfast	Stovetop oatmeal porridge with blueberries
Lunch	Cottage cheese and tomato bagel
Dinner	Lentil and veggie soup
Snack	Carrot sticks and home-made hummus

Wednesday	
Breakfast	Fruit and veggie smoothie
Lunch	Lentil and veggie soup
Dinner	Vegetable tacos with cilantro sauce
Snack	Apple and peanut butter stacks

Thursday	
Breakfast	Oatmeal with cinnamon and raisins
Lunch	Vegetable tacos with cilantro sauce
Dinner	Zucchini "zoodles" with parmesan
Snack	Toast with almond butter and banana

Friday	
Breakfast	Avocado toast with poached eggs
Lunch	Quick black bean salad
Dinner	Vegetarian one-pot chili
Snack	Peanut butter and celery snack

Saturday	
Breakfast	Loaded vegetable omelet
Lunch	Vegetarian one-pot chili
Dinner	Zucchini "zoodles" with parmesan
Snack	Mixed berries and yogurt
Sunday	
Breakfast	Oatmeal with cinnamon and raisins
Lunch	Whole wheat feta and veggie sandwich
Dinner	Vegetable tacos with cilantro sauce
Snack	Granola and berries bowl

MEAL PLAN WEEK 3

Day	Meals
Monday	
Breakfast	Avocado toast with poached eggs
Lunch	Zucchini "zoodles" with parmesan
Dinner	Lentil and veggie soup
Snack	Carrot sticks and home-made hummus

Tuesday	
Breakfast	Loaded vegetable omelet
Lunch	Lentil and veggie soup
Dinner	Vegetarian one-pot chili
Snack	Granola and berries bowl

Wednesday	
Breakfast	Fruit and nuts breakfast bowl
Lunch	Vegetarian one-pot chili
Dinner	Quick black bean salad
Snack	Blueberry banana smoothie

Thursday	
Breakfast	Oatmeal with cinnamon and raisins
Lunch	Chickpea and quinoa bowl
Dinner	Thai pumpkin curry
Snack	Peanut butter and celery snack

Friday	
Breakfast	Stovetop oatmeal porridge with blueberries
Lunch	Cottage cheese and tomato bagel
Dinner	Lentil and veggie soup
Snack	Toast with almond butter and banana

Saturday	
Breakfast	Oatmeal with cinnamon and raisins
Lunch	Whole wheat feta and veggie sandwich
Dinner	Vegetable tacos with cilantro sauce
Snack	Mixed berries and yogurt
Sunday	
Breakfast	Loaded vegetable omelet
Lunch	Vegetable tacos with cilantro sauce
Dinner	Zucchini "zoodles" with parmesan
Snack	Apple and peanut butter stacks

9

RECIPES FOR BREAKFAST

LOADED VEGETABLE OMELET

Prep Time: 5 minutes

Cook Time: 10 minutes

Servings: 1

Ingredients

- 1 zucchini, grated
- 1 oz frozen peas
- 1 handful cherry tomatoes, halved
- 1 handful fresh kale
- 1 pinch dried chili flakes
- 1 sliced garlic clove, large
- 2 eggs, beaten well

- ½ tbsp white wine vinegar
- 2 tsp olive oil
- A drizzle of olive oil to fry the omelet
- Sand pepper to taste
- Seasoning spices and herbs of preference for the cherry tomatoes

Instructions

1. Place the halved cherry tomatoes into a bowl, drizzle with the white wine vinegar, and sprinkle with the seasoning of our choice, then set the bowl aside.
2. Place the eggs into a small mixing bowl and beat well. Add salt and pepper if using and mix through. Set the bowl aside.
3. Heat the olive oil in a small frying pan, add the garlic and cook until fragrant for about 1 minute. Add the grated zucchini and cook until all the liquid has evaporated for about 5 minutes.
4. Add the peas and the kale and continue cooking until the kale is wilted for about 2 minutes.
5. Add the chili flakes, and season the mixture with any herbs of your preference. Add salt

and pepper to taste and stir the mixture to combine.

6. Place a small, nonstick frying pan on the head and add a drizzle of olive oil. Add the beaten eggs and swirl the pan to ensure the egg mixture is distributed evenly.

7. Check the bottom of the omelet by lifting the sides, and once it is brown, scoop the cooked vegetables onto half of the omelet, then gently fold the other half over the vegetables.

8. Please note to not cook the omelet on too high of heat, as the bottom will brown too fast. The top of the omelet must be nearly cooked by the time the bottom has browned.

9. Place the omelet on a plate using a spatula and place the cherry tomatoes next to the omelet on the plate. Serve warm.

Nutritional Facts/Info per Serving: *Calories 307; Carbs 8.4 g; Fat 19.2 g;Protein 22.4 g*

FRUIT AND VEGGIE SMOOTHIE

Prep Time: 5 minutes

Cook Time: 0 minutes

Servings: 1

Ingredients

- ½ cup sliced blueberries, or strawberries, or mango, chopped
- 1 fresh or frozen medium banana
- 1 tbsp almond butter
- ½ cup almond milk, unsweetened
- ¼ cup plain low-fat Greek yogurt
- ½ cup baby spinach

Instructions

1. Place all the ingredients into a blender and blend until perfectly smooth.
2. If the smoothie is too thick, add a splash of almond milk; if the consistency is too thin, add a few ice cubes and blend for a few seconds.
3. Serve immediately or place in the fridge to use later.

Notes

1. Optional extras to add before blending are any of the following:

2. ½ tsp ginger, peeled and chopped.
3. 2–3 mint leaves.
4. 1–2 basil leaves.
5. For a nut-free smoothie, replace the almond butter with any of the following:
6. Pumpkin seeds
7. Ground flax seeds
8. Sunflower seeds
9. Replace the Greek yogurt with coconut milk yogurt for a dairy-free smoothie.

Nutritional Facts/Info per Serving: *Calories 300; Carbs 40 g; Fat 11g; Protein 12.5 g*

AVOCADO TOAST WITH POACHED EGGS

Prep Time: 5 minutes

Cook Time: 5 minutes

Servings: 1

Ingredients

- 2 slices whole grain bread
- 2 tbsp Parmesan cheese, shaved
- 2 eggs

- fresh chopped herbs of choice for topping such as thyme, parsley, or basil
- 1 tomato, quartered
- ⅓ avocado
- Salt and pepper to taste

Instructions

1. Place a deep, nonstick frying pan on medium heat and pour enough water into the pan so that it will cover the eggs when poaching (roughly 1 inch of water). When the water boils, place two mason jar metal outer rims in the pan. Turn the heat off once the water is boiling rapidly.
2. Carefully crack 1 egg into each of the mason jar rings. Place a lid on the pan and poach the eggs as follows:
3. 4 minutes for very soft and runny yolks.
4. 4 ½ minutes for soft yolks.
5. 5 or more minutes for semi-soft yolks.
6. Toast the bread and mash the avocado while the eggs are poaching. Divide the mashed avocado between the two slices of toast and spread the avocado over the toast.
7. Once the eggs are done, remove them (still in

the rims) from the water, using a spatula, and place on a clean plate. Then, gently remove the metal rims from the eggs and place an egg on top of the avocado on the toast.

8. Sprinkle the eggs with salt and pepper and top with the Parmesan shavings.

9. Garnish the eggs with the chopped herbs, place the quartered tomato next to the toast, and serve immediately.

Nutritional Facts/Info per Serving: *Calories 393; Carbs 30.1 g; Fat 20.4 g; Protein 23.3 g*

OATMEAL WITH CINNAMON AND RAISINS

Prep Time: 2 minutes

Cook Time: 10 minutes

Servings: 1

Ingredients

- ½ cup rolled oats
- 1 tbsp raisins
- ½ banana, sliced (put a few slices aside for garnish)
- 1 cup of nondairy milk or water (see notes)

- 1 tbsp coconut butter
- 1 tsp cinnamon
- ½ tbsp ground flax seeds (optional)
- 1 tsp maple syrup (optional)
- Pinch of salt

Instructions

1. Place a pot on the stove on medium-high heat and add the water or nondairy milk.
2. Add the oats, raisins, banana slices, cinnamon, flax seed, and salt to the pot and stir.
3. Cook on medium-high heat until all the liquid has been absorbed into the porridge. Stir the porridge a few times during cooking to ensure that the banana slices break up in the oats. The oatmeal is ready when it has thickened.
4. Spoon the oats into a bowl and place the reserved banana sliced on top. Add the maple syrup and coconut butter on top of the banana slices, and lastly, sprinkle with cinnamon.
5. Serve warm.

Notes

1. You can use just nondairy milk, just water, or a blend of water and milk for this recipe.
2. Any nondairy milk is suitable to use.
3. Nut or seed butter of your preference can be substituted for coconut butter.

Nutritional Facts/Info per Serving: *Calories 484; Carbs 62 g; Fat 22 g;Protein 14g*

FRUIT AND NUTS BREAKFAST BOWL

Prep Time: 10 minutes

Cook Time: 0 minutes

Servings: 1 (1 ⅓ cup)

Ingredients

- ⅔ cup raspberries, frozen
- ¼ cup blueberries
- ½ frozen banana slices
- 5 tbsp almonds sliced and divided
- ½ cup plain almond milk, unsweetened
- 1 tbsp coconut flakes, unsweetened
- ¼ tsp cinnamon, ground

- ⅛ tsp vanilla extract
- ⅛ tsp cardamom, ground

Instructions

1. Place the almond milk, raspberries, 3 tablespoons of the almonds, banana, cardamom, vanilla, and cinnamon in a blender and blend until the mixture is perfectly smooth.
2. Pour the mixture into a serving bowl and top with the coconut flakes, the remaining 2 tablespoons of almonds, and the blueberries.
3. Serve immediately or place in a suitable airtight container in the fridge.

Nutritional Facts/Info per Serving: *Calories 360; Carbs 45.6 g;Fat 19 g; Protein 9.2 g*

STOVETOP OATMEAL PORRIDGE WITH BLUEBERRIES

Prep Time: 2 minutes

Cook Time: 7 minutes

Servings: 3

Ingredients

- 1 cup milk
- 2 cups rolled oats
- 2 ½ cups water
- 1 ½ cups fresh blueberries
- ½ tsp vanilla extract (optional)
- 2 tbsp honey, or less as to preference

Instructions

1. Wash the blueberries and set them aside.
2. Place the oats, milk, and water into a saucepan and mix thoroughly.
3. Bring the mixture to a boil and then reduce the heat down to medium.
4. Cook the porridge until the oats are soft and nearly cooked. Stir the porridge frequently to prevent the oats from sticking to the bottom of the saucepan.
5. Add the blueberries and stir well. Continue cooking the porridge until the oats are completely soft, and the blueberries have started to soften. Using a fork, mash some of the blueberries to distribute the flavor throughout the oats.

6. Add the vanilla extract and honey to the porridge and stir to combine.
7. Serve the porridge warm.

Notes

- The cooked porridge can be stored in airtight containers in the fridge for 4–6 days.
- Stevia or maple syrup can be substituted for honey.
- Optional ingredients such as ground cardamom and cinnamon can be added for a spicy flavor.
- Frozen blueberries can be used instead of fresh.

Nutritional Facts/Info per Serving: *Calories 340, Carbs 69 g; Fat 4 g; Protein 10 g*

RECIPES FOR LUNCH

WHOLE WHEAT FETA AND VEGGIE SANDWICH

Prep Time: 3 minutes

Cook Time: 0 minutes

Servings: 1

Ingredients

- 2 slices whole wheat bread
- 2 tbsp Feta cheese, crumbled
- ¼ cup sprouts of own preference
- 2 chopped peppadew peppers
- 3 tbsp cilantro jalapeño hummus (see notes)
- 1 fresh lettuce leaf

- 1 small red onion, sliced
- 2 slices cucumber
- 2 slices tomato

Instructions

1. Toast the bread if preferred or use it untoasted.
2. Spread the hummus evenly over both slices of bread and then layer the rest of the ingredients on one slice, placing the other slice of bread on top.
3. Slice the sandwich in half and serve immediately.

Notes

1. If the sandwich will be eaten later, it is preferable to pack the prepared ingredients in an airtight container and then assemble the sandwich when ready to eat. Assembling it well ahead of time can result in the vegetables becoming soggy.
2. Regular or sweet and spicy hummus can be substituted for the cilantro jalapeño hummus.

Nutritional Facts/Info per Serving: *Calories 365 Carbs 49.9 g;Fat 14.3 g; Protein 10.5 g*

COTTAGE CHEESE AND TOMATO BAGEL

Prep Time: 4 minutes

Cook Time: 0 minutes

Servings: 1

Ingredients

- 1 bagel, whole grain (preferred)
- 6 oz cottage cheese, low-fat
- 4 slices tomato
- 1 tbsp fresh chives, chopped
- 1 minced clove garlic
- Salt and pepper to taste
- Assorted fresh herbs for garnish (optional)

Instructions

1. Place the cottage cheese, chives, garlic, salt, and pepper into a food processor and pulse until the mixture is smooth.
2. Spread the mixture on the bagel, top with

the tomato slices, and add the optional fresh herbs if using.

3. Serve immediately or place in the fridge in an airtight container to serve later.

Nutritional Facts/Info per Serving: *Calories 367.8; Carbs 55.8 g; Fat 4g, Protein 31.8 g*

CHICKPEA AND QUINOA BOWLS

Prep Time: 20 minutes

Cook Time: 0 minutes

Servings: 4 (1 ½ cup per serving)

Ingredients

- 2 cups quinoa, cooked
- 1 can (15 oz) chickpeas, rinsed
- ¼ cup Feta cheese, crumbled
- ¼ cup chopped Kalamata olives
- 4 tbsp olive oil, divided
- 1 jar (7 oz) roasted red peppers, rinsed
- 1 cup cucumber, diced
- ¼ cup red onion, finely chopped
- ¼ cup almonds, slivered
- 2 tbsp fresh parsley, finely chopped

- 1 garlic clove, minced
- ½ tsp ground cumin
- 1 tsp paprika
- ¼ tsp crushed red pepper (optional)

Instructions

1. Put 2 tablespoons of olive oil, red peppers, paprika, almonds, cumin, garlic, and crushed red peppers (if you use this) into a food processor or blender and purée until the mixture is mostly smooth.
2. Put the quinoa, chickpeas, red onion, remaining 2 tablespoons of olive oil, and olives into a medium-sized mixing bowl and stir to combine.
3. Divide the quinoa mixture equally among 4 bowls and top each bowl with equal amounts of red pepper purée and cucumber. Sprinkle the Feta cheese and parsley on top and serve.

Notes

1. This recipe is a great meal prep lunch to eat at home or to take to work (I skip the onions if I take it to work though…).

2. Cook the quinoa and make the red pepper purée in advance to store it in separate containers in the fridge.

3. Prepare the other vegetables and store them in separate containers, and then assemble the salad just before serving.

Nutritional Facts/Info per Serving: *Calories 479; Carbs 49.5 g;Fat 24.8;Protein 12.7 g*

QUICK BLACK BEAN SALAD

Prep Time: 30 minutes

Cook Time: 0 minutes

Servings: 4 (2 cups per serving)

Ingredients

- 1 can (15 oz) black beans, rinsed
- 2 cups (10 oz) grape tomatoes, halved
- 8 cups salad greens, mixed
- 2 cups frozen corn thawed and patted dry (see notes)
- 1 ripe medium avocado, pitted and chopped into chunks
- ½ cup red onion, thinly sliced

- 2 tbsp olive oil
- ¼ cup fresh cilantro leaves
- ¼ cup lime juice
- 1 minced garlic clove
- ½ tsp salt

Instructions

1. Place the sliced red onion into a small bowl and cover with cold water. Set the bowl aside.
2. Put the avocado, lime juice, cilantro, garlic, olive oil, and salt into a food processor or blender and purée until the mixture is creamy and smooth. Scrape the sides of the blender or food processor clean if needed to ensure the purée is fully combined.
3. When ready to serve, place the salad greens, black beans, and corn into a large mixing bowl. Drain the water off the onion and add onion. Lastly, add the avocado purée and toss the salad lightly.
4. Divide the salad equally between 4 bowls or plates and serve.

Notes

1. Canned corn or the corn kernels from two fresh ears of corn can be used instead of frozen corn.
2. If making this salad ahead of time, prepare the salad ingredients and store each ingredient in a separate airtight container in the fridge. Do not prepare the avocado purée ahead of time; prepare this when you are ready to serve the black bean salad.

Nutritional Facts/Info per Serving: *Calories 322; Carbs 40.8 g; Fat 16 g; Protein 10.6 g*

11

RECIPES FOR DINNER

ZUCCHINI ZOODLES WITH PARMESAN

Prep Time: 8 minutes

Cook Time: 12 minutes

Servings: 4

Ingredients

- 32 oz (2 lb) zucchini (roughly 4 medium)
- ½ cup parmesan cheese, plus extra for garnish
- 12 oz (2 medium) tomatoes, chopped
- 3 tbsp olive oil
- ¼–½ tsp crushed red pepper flakes (according to personal spicy preference)

- 1 tbsp minced garlic
- 1 tsp cornstarch
- 1 cup torn fresh basil leaves
- 2 tsp cold water
- Salt to taste

Instructions

1. Wash and dry the zucchini and spiralize them. Cut the noodles to about the length of spaghetti (see notes).
2. Place a large, deep skillet on the stove on medium heat and add the olive oil, red pepper flakes, and garlic. Add the zucchini noodles when the oil starts to bubble. Use pasta tongs to toss the noodles and cook for 5–7 minutes until the noodles are al dente.
3. Take care not to overcook the noodles. They must be wilted but still be crunchy, so do not cook them longer than 7 minutes, or they will become mushy. Keep tossing the noodles while it cooks so that they cook evenly.
4. Stir in the tomatoes, Parmesan cheese, and basil and continue cooking for 1 minute. Remove the noodle mixture from the skillet

with pasta tongs, allowing the liquid to drip out into the skillet. Place noodles into a serving dish and set the dish aside.

5. Heat the liquid in the skillet until it starts to simmer. Combine the cornstarch and cold water in a small mixing bowl and add it to the simmering liquid. Keep whisking and cook for 1 minute until the sauce thickens. Add the salt to the sauce and adjust the seasoning if necessary.

6. Pour the sauce over the noodles mixture and add more Parmesan cheese as garnish.

7. Divide the noodles equally into 4 portions and serve immediately.

Notes

1. If you do not have a spiralizer, use a vegetable peeler to make ribbon or wide noodles, or use a mandoline or julienne vegetable peeler to make the noodles by hand.

2. It is normal for the liquid to settle in the bottom of bowls during eating so just blend the liquid into the mixture with a fork.

3. The Parmesan cheese can be substituted

with any hard cheese that is vegetarian-friendly. To make the dish vegan, replace the cheese with nutritional yeast, starting with 2 tablespoons of yeast until it is to your taste.

Nutritional Facts/Info per Serving:*Calories 197, Carbs 11.2 g; Fat 14.3 g; Protein 19.7 g*

VEGETABLE TACOS WITH CILANTRO SAUCE

Prep Time: 20 minutes

Cook Time: 25 minutes

Servings: 6 (2 tacos plus 1 tbsp of sauce per serving)

Ingredients for Tacos

- 12 medium or 24 small flour or corn tortillas
- 1 can (15 oz) black beans, drained and rinsed, or 1 ½ cups cooked black beans
- 10 cherry tomatoes, halved
- ½ medium red onion, cut into 1/4 -inch blocks
- 1 medium avocado, cubed
- Pickled red onions (optional)
- 1 seeded red bell pepper, cut into ¼-inch blocks

- 1 medium zucchini, cut into ¼-inch blocks
- 2 tsp chili powder
- 1 tbsp olive oil
- Salt to taste

Ingredients for Cilantro Sauce

- ½ cup sour cream
- ½ jalapeño chili pepper, membranes, and seeds removed
- ½ cup cilantro stems and leaves, tightly packed
- 2 tbsp lime juice, fresh
- Salt to taste

Instructions

1. Heat the oven to 425 °F and line a baking sheet with aluminum foil or parchment paper.
2. Prepare the vegetables and then place the bell pepper, zucchini, tomatoes, and onion on the baking sheet. Drizzle the vegetables with olive oil and sprinkle ¾ of a teaspoon of chili powder and 2 or 4 pinches of salt over the vegetables. Toss the vegetables

with two spoons to coat them in the seasoning.

3. Roast the vegetables for 25 minutes until they are tender, stirring the vegetables a few times during the baking to ensure they roast evenly.

4. Remove the baking sheet from the oven about 5 minutes before the vegetables are fully roasted. Toss the black beans with a drizzle of olive oil and ¼ teaspoon of chili powder and add the beans to the baking sheet. Put the baking sheet back in the oven and continue roasting until the veggies are tender and fully done, and the beans are hot.

5. Make the cilantro sauce while the vegetables are roasting. Put the sour cream, jalapeño, lime juice, cilantro, and a pinch of salt in a blender and pulse until the mixture is smooth. Taste and adjust the salt and lime juice to your taste. Pour the cilantro sauce into a suitable container with a lid and set it aside.

6. Place the tortillas in two stacks and wrap each stack in aluminum foil. Place the stacks into the oven until they are heated through for about 10–15 minutes.

7. Fill each tortilla equally with the vegetable and beans mixture. Top each filled tortilla with pickled onions and avocado, and lastly, drizzle a ½ tablespoon of cilantro sauce over the top of each taco.

8. Serve warm.

Notes

1. The beans and vegetable mixture can be made well in advance and then reheated; the tacos can be assembled as and when needed. The roasted filling can be stored in the fridge for up to a week.

2. The cilantro sauce will also stay fresh in the fridge for up to a week.

3. The sour cream can be substituted with tahini to make this cilantro sauce vegan.

Nutritional Facts/Info per Serving: *Calories 286; Carbs 42 g Fat 11 g Protein 9 g*

CAULIFLOWER STEAKS WITH CHIMICHURRI SAUCE

Prep Time: 15 minutes

Cook Time: 20 minutes

Servings: 2 (½ of the dish- 2 steaks - plus 2 tbsp chimichurri sauce per serving)

Ingredients for Cauliflower Steaks

- 1 head of cauliflower, medium-sized
- Salt and pepper to taste
- 2–3 tbsp olive oil

Ingredients for Chimichurri Sauce

- 1 medium shallot
- 2 cups of tightly packed parsley, stems, and leaves
- ½ to 1 tsp crushed red pepper flakes (see notes)
- ⅓ cup red wine vinegar
- 1 tbsp minced garlic
- ½ cup olive oil
- ½ to ¾ tsp salt

Instructions

1. Place the shallots and garlic in a blender or processor and pulse until minced. Add the red pepper flakes, salt, and parsley, and pulse until the ingredients are chopped small.
2. Scrape the sides clean and add the red wine vinegar and oil. Pulse for 30 seconds or until the sauce is blended.
3. Taste and add salt and red pepper flakes to your taste. Pour the sauce into a suitable container and set it aside.
4. Heat up the oven to 400 °F.
5. Wash the head of cauliflower and remove any outer leaves. Trip the stem, but leave enough to create a solid, flat base, and cut the cauliflower in half from the top to the stem.
6. Create cauliflower steaks by trimming the rounded edges of the cauliflower to create 1 ½–2-inch thick steaks (4 steaks) that still have a stem attached to them. It is important to keep some of the stems attached to each steak, as this will prevent them from falling apart.
7. Heat the olive oil to medium heat in an

ovenproof skillet that is large enough to take the 4 steaks. Cook the steaks for about 5 minutes until golden brown. Then, carefully flip the steaks over using a spatula and continue cooking for another 3–5 minutes until browned. Occasionally lift the steaks during the cooking time to ensure that the oil coats the bottom of the pan.

8. Season the steaks with salt and any optional condiments you wish to use after you have turned the steaks over.

9. If you do not have an ovenproof skillet large enough to accommodate all 4 steaks, then use a normal skillet. After the steaks have been browned on both sides, carefully remove the steaks and place them on a baking sheet lined with aluminum foil or parchment paper. A silicone baking mat can also be used for roasting the steaks in the oven.

10. Place the ovenproof skillet in the oven and roast for 8–10 minutes. The steaks are done when they can be pierced with a fork, and the stems are tender.

11. Garnish each of the steaks with 1 tablespoon of chimichurri sauce and serve them warm

with any of the optional serving suggestions and toppings.

Notes

1. Leftover chimichurri sauce can be stored in the fridge for 3 or 4 days in an airtight container. The vibrant green color of the parsley may fade slightly, but that does not affect the taste.
2. The best way to store prepared chimichurri sauce to have prepared sauce on hand is to freeze it in single portions in ice trays and then transfer them to freezer bags. The sauce can be stored in the freezer for up to 3 months.
3. Do not discard the cauliflower that has been trimmed from the head, as it can be used to make mashed cauliflower and cauliflower rice.

Nutritional Facts/Info per Serving: *Calories 325; Carbs 16.6 g; Fat 28.8 g; Protein 6.6 g*

LENTIL AND VEGGIE SOUP

Prep Time: 10 minutes

Cook Time: 50 minutes

Servings: 6

Ingredients

- 2 cups (12 oz) picked and rinsed lentils
- 2 cups onion, finely chopped
- 2 heaped cups of spinach or kale, shredded
- 1 ½ cups carrots, chopped
- 8 cups of vegetable or chicken broth
- 2 tbsp olive oil
- 2 tsp minced garlic
- ½ tsp ground coriander
- ½ tsp ground turmeric
- 1 tsp ground cumin
- ½ tsp ground black pepper
- Salt to taste
- 1–2 lemons
- ¼ of fresh herbs of your choice, chopped (optional)

Instructions

1. Place a large pot (a deep cast-iron pot works great) on the stovetop on medium heat. Add the oil, and when heated, add the carrot, onions, and ¼ teaspoon of salt and cook for about 5–7 minutes, stirring a few times until the onions start to smell sweet and have softened. Add the garlic, coriander, cumin, turmeric, and black pepper and cook for 30 seconds while stirring.

2. Increase the heat to high and add the broth and the lentils to the pot and bring it to boiling point. Taste and adjust the salt by adding ½ to 1 teaspoon to your preference. Reduce the heat and cook on simmer for 35–40 minutes with a lid partially covering the pot. Test to see if the lentils are tender, and if not, cook for a few additional minutes.

3. Add the spinach or kale and cook for 5 minutes with the pot uncovered. Remove the pot from the heat and stir in the fresh herbs and the juice of half a lemon. Taste the soup again and add additional seasoning, lemon juice, and salt if needed.

4. The soup is ready to serve, or if you prefer a

smooth soup, blend it to your preferred consistency with an immersion blender. Alternatively, blend half the soup in a standard blender, then return it to the pot and stir through.

Notes

1. The soup can be stored in the fridge for up to 4 days and then reheated as needed.
2. The soup can be frozen for 4–5 minutes in airtight containers and reheated from frozen in the microwave on the stovetop.
3. If you find the soup too thick when reheating it, add water or broth a few spoons at a time until you have the desired consistency.

Nutritional Facts/Info per Serving: *Calories 298; Carbs 45.3 g; Fat 5.5 g; Protein 19.5 g*

THAI PUMPKIN CURRY

Prep Time: 15 minutes

Cook Time: 30 minutes

Servings: 4

Ingredients

- 3 ½ cups butternut squash or pumpkin, peeled and cubed
- 1 cup broccoli, chopped
- 1 minced shallot, medium size
- 1 large thinly sliced lengthwise red bell pepper
- ⅔ cup roasted cashews, unsalted or lightly salted
- 1 small thinly sliced serrano or red chili, stems and seeds removed
- 1 ½ tbsp coconut oil (see notes)
- 2 cans (14 oz each) light coconut milk (see notes for alternatives)
- 3 tbsp red or yellow Thai curry paste
- 1 tbsp coconut aminos
- 2 tbsp lemon juice
- 2 tbsp finely minced garlic
- 2 tbsp fresh minced ginger
- 1 tsp ground turmeric
- 2 tbsp coconut sugar or maple syrup (can be substituted with Stevia)
- ¼ tsp salt
- Fresh cilantro or basil for garnish (optional)

- Lemon juice for garnish (optional)

Instructions

1. Place a large pot on the stovetop on medium heat. When the pot is hot, add the coconut oil, pepper, shallot, garlic, and ginger. Sauté the mixture for 2–3 minutes while stirring.
2. Add the curry paste and bell pepper and continue cooking for another 2 minutes. Add the pumpkin and cook for another 2 minutes, stirring occasionally.
3. Add coconut milk, coconut aminos, turmeric, coconut sugar or maple syrup, and salt. Stir to mix the ingredients and then bring the pot to a simmer on medium heat.
4. Once the food is simmering, turn the heat to low and place a lid on the pot. It is important not to boil the food but to keep it simmering.
5. Cook for 10–15 minutes to allow the pumpkin to absorb the curry flavor and soften.
6. Taste the broth during the cooking time and adjust the salt and seasonings to taste; add extra curry paste as per personal preference.
7. Once the pumpkin is tender and the broth

seasoned to your taste, add the lemon juice, broccoli, and cashews. Place a lid on the pot and simmer on medium-low heat for 3–4 minutes.

8. Garnish with fresh cilantro or basil leaves and lemon juice (optional).

9. Serve the curry warm with any of the serving suggestions in the notes.

Notes

1. If you prefer very thick and creamy curry, then scoop out half of the sauce/broth and half of the pumpkin once the curry is done, and put it into a blender, blending until smooth. Try not to include any of the broccoli pieces when blending. Return the blended vegetables to the curry pot, stir, and warm through.

2. Serve the pumpkin with brown rice, cauliflower rice, or coconut quinoa. (Please note the serving options are not calculated into the nutritional values).

3. Grapeseed oil or avocado oil can be substituted for the coconut oil in this recipe.

If you are avoiding oil, use water instead of oil.

4. If you want an extra creamy sauce, use full-fat coconut milk. This will slightly increase the macros.

5. If a thinner curry sauce is preferred, use a can of coconut milk and an equal amount of vegetable broth.

6. The coconut aminos can be substituted with soy sauce or tamari sauce for a non-gluten-free option.

7. The cooked Thai pumpkin curry can be stored in the fridge for 3 or 4 days in an airtight container and can be frozen for up to a month. Reheat in the microwave or on the stovetop.

Nutritional Facts/Info per Serving: *Calories 423; Carbs 39.9 g; Fat 29.1 g; Protein 9.1 g*

VEGETARIAN ONE-POT CHILI

Prep Time: 15 minutes

Cook Time: 40 minutes

Servings: 6 (1 ½ cups per serving)

Ingredients

- 2 cans (15 oz each) white or kidney beans
- 2 cans (28 oz each) whole tomatoes
- 2 diced carrots, medium
- 2 diced bell peppers
- 2 cups corn, frozen
- 3 diced celery stalks
- 1 large onion, diced
- 4 finely minced garlic cloves
- 2 tbsp olive oil
- 2 tbsp cumin
- 1–3 tbsp chili powder
- 1 tsp oregano
- ¼–2 tsp crushed chili flakes (adjust as to preference)
- 2 tsp salt or to taste

Instructions

1. Place a large pot on the stovetop on medium-high heat; then, add the oil. Add the onion and sauté for 2–3 minutes. Add the garlic and continue to sauté for 1 minute. Add the cumin, chili flakes, oregano, and chili powder and stir the mix for 30 seconds.

2. Add the celery, peppers, and carrots and cook until the vegetables start to soften for about 5 minutes.

3. Pour the tomatoes into a bowl and crush them using your hand. Add the tomatoes with the juice to the pot and bring the mixture in the pot to a simmer.

4. Reduce the heat down to medium-low and let the chili simmer for 20 minutes with no lid on the pot. Stir the chili from time to time to prevent it from sticking to the bottom of the pot.

5. After 20 minutes, add the corn and the beans and bring the pot back to a simmer. Continue simmering until the beans and the corn have heated through for about 5 minutes.

6. Taste and add salt as per personal preference.

7. Serve the chili warm as it is, or add any of the optional toppings and serving suggestion items in the notes.

Notes

1. You can add any of these optional toppings

and with any of the serving suggestions, taking into account that these items are not calculated into the macros for the chili.

2. Toppings:
3. Diced avocado
4. Sour cream
5. Greek yogurt
6. Chopped red pickled onions
7. Chopped fresh cilantro
8. Sliced green onions
9. Sprinkle nutritional yeast over the chili for an extra cheesy taste.
10. Serving ideas:
11. Whole wheat soda bread
12. Cornbread
13. Zucchini cornbread muffins
14. Brown rice
15. This chili can be stored in the fridge for up to 4 days in an airtight container and frozen for 4–6 months.

RECIPES FOR SNACKS

APPLE AND PEANUT BUTTER STACKS

Prep Time: 5 minutes

Cook Time: 0 minutes

Servings: 1

Ingredients

- 1 apple, type of your choice
- 1 tbsp natural peanut butter or other nut butter of choice

Instructions

1. Place an apple corer on top of the apple and

firmly press down, twisting the corer until it goes through the bottom of the apple, and then remove the corer.

2. You can use the apple without removing the skin. Place it on its side on a cutting board and slice the apple into 6 evenly sized apple rings.

3. Put 1 teaspoon of peanut butter on each of 3 slices and spread over the slices; then, place the remaining 3 slices on top of each slice with peanut butter.

4. Serve immediately.

5. If making the apple stack ahead of serving, rub a small amount of lemon juice over the slices to prevent them from turning brown.

Nutritional Facts/Info per Serving:

Calories 175; Carbs 30 g, Fat 8 g, Protein 7 g

MIXED BERRIES WITH YOGURT

Prep Time: 5 minutes

Cook Time: 0 minutes

Servings: 1

Ingredients

- 1 cup fresh strawberries, chopped
- ½ cup blueberries
- ¾ cup plain Greek yogurt
- 1 tbsp honey

Instructions

1. Wash the berries and set them aside to dry.
2. Place the yogurt in a serving bowl and add the berries on top.
3. Drizzle the honey over the berries and serve.

Nutritional Facts/Info per Serving:

Calories 240; Carbs 44 g; Fat 1 g; Protein 16 g

GRANOLA AND BERRIES BOWL

Prep Time: 10 minutes

Cook Time: 0 minutes

Servings: 1

Ingredients

- ½ cup mixed berries (strawberries, blueberries, raspberries, and blackberries)
- ¾ cup Greek yogurt (honey vanilla flavor)
- 3 tbsp granola
- 2 tbsp sliced almonds

Instructions

1. Put the yogurt into a small serving bowl then add the berries.
2. Top with granola and nuts.
3. Serve immediately.

Notes

1. Optional extras, not calculated in the macros, can be added, such as:
2. 1 teaspoon of chia seeds: Take note that chia seeds absorb liquid fast, so if using, add them when you are ready to serve.
3. Drizzle pure maple syrup or honey over the granola or sprinkle 1 teaspoon of sweetener of your choice over the yogurt.

Nutritional Facts/Info per Serving:

Calories 206; Carbs 21.3 g; Fat 7 g; Protein 16.4 g

BLUEBERRY BANANA SMOOTHIE

Prep Time: 5 minutes

Cook Time: 0 minutes

Servings: 2

Ingredients

- ½ cup Greek yogurt
- 2 cups coconut water
- 1 frozen banana
- 2 cups frozen blueberries
- 1 tbsp flax seeds

Instructions

1. Blend all the ingredients in a blender on high speed until creamy for about 30 seconds.
2. Divide smoothie mixture into 2 equal portions and serve.

Notes

1. Leftover smoothie mixture can be stored in the refrigerator for around 2 days.
2. If you have fresh blueberries, it is best to freeze them for a few hours before making the smoothie.
3. Dairy-free coconut yogurt can be substituted for Greek yogurt.

Nutritional Facts/Info per Serving:

Calories 238; Carbs 47 g; Fat 3 g, Protein 9 g

TOAST WITH ALMOND BUTTER AND BANANA

Prep Time: 5 minutes

Cook Time: 0 minutes

Servings: 1

Ingredients

- 1 slice toasted rye bread
- 1 tbsp almond butter
- 1 sliced banana

Instructions

1. Toast the bread and spread almond butter evenly on it.
2. Top with the sliced banana and serve immediately.

Nutritional Facts/Info per Serving:

Calories 280; Carbs 44 g; Fat 11 g; Protein 6 g

PEANUT BUTTER AND CELERY SNACK

Prep Time: 5 minutes

Cook Time: 0 minutes

Servings: 1

Ingredients

- 2 tbsp peanut butter
- 2 celery stalks, medium

Instructions

1. Rinse and clean the celery stalks and cut them into 2-inch pieces.

2. Spread the peanut butter evenly into the celery pieces and serve.

Notes

1. Two tablespoons of peanut butter powder can be substituted for the peanut butter. Please note that the calories per serving will change as peanut butter powder is much lower in calories:
2. *Calories* 84
3. *Carbs* 6 g
4. *Fat* 0 g
5. *Protein* 6 g
6. The following optional extras, that are not included in the nutritional values, can be added:
7. Small pieces of dried fruit or freeze-dried fruit
8. A sprinkling of coconut over the pieces of celery
9. A sprinkling of cereal or granola on top of the celery pieces
10. Nuts and seeds such as sesame seeds, sunflower seeds, chia seeds, and crushed peanuts

Nutritional Facts/Info per Serving: *Calories 216; Carbs 5.4 g; Fat 18 g; Protein 12 g*

CARROT STICKS WITH CHICKPEA HUMMUS

Prep Time: 2 minutes

Cook Time: 0 minutes

Servings: 1

Ingredients

- 1 (4 ½ oz) large carrot
- 3 tbsp chickpea hummus (suggested brand is Sabra)

Instructions

1. Peel the carrot and cut it into sticks.
2. Put the hummus into a small bowl.
3. Serve at room temperature.

Nutritional Facts/Info per Serving: *Calories 171; Carbs 9 g; Fat 11 g; Protein 6 g*

13

FREE AND ALMOST-FREE FOOD

CAN FOOD REALLY BE FREE?

Let's face it: When you think about the word "diet,"
the idea of meager portions and constant hunger
comes to mind. That's one of the things that makes
dieting feel like your own personal purgatory and
creates the concept of a diet being something you
have to suffer through. This concept of suffering
triggers our desire for instant gratification. We want
to lose as much weight as possible in as short a
period as possible, so we don't have to experience
the unpleasantness of the hunger and cravings typically associated with dieting. We need to change that
idea as a way of mentally accepting a healthy diet as

a long-term goal. It's part of what we discussed under the chapter on the first day of preparation.

When you accept a healthy diet as a long-term goal, you accept it as a way of life and start to shift away from the idea of crash dieting and the tendency to yo-yo diet. However, just because you are following a healthy diet (that doesn't dramatically slash your daily calories to half-starve yourself thin) doesn't mean you shouldn't keep an eye on your daily caloric intake. This is where free food comes in.

Have you heard the terms "free food" or "almost-free food" before? No, it doesn't mean getting food without having to pay for it. Free food and almost-free food, in the healthy eating world, is food that allows you to fill up without breaking your daily calorie budget. Free and almost-free food can be misleading, but when you think about it, if you can fill up on the "cheap," you can stick to your diet without being left feeling hungry and deprived. So what exactly is free and almost-free food, and how does it work? Well, buckle up because you're about to get a crash course on how to use free and almost-free food as your "Get Out of Jail Free" card!

HOW DOES IT WORK?

Free food isn't technically free, per se. It does cost something, but that cost is extremely low. It refers to non-starchy vegetables that are high in fiber and fairly low in carbohydrates and calories. You can eat as much of these vegetables as you like without running up your calorie bill too high for the day. "Wait, what? Are you saying I can eat as much as I want? Cool! Fried jalapeño poppers, tempura fried broccoli, and stuffed mushrooms, here I come!" Right?

Not quite. While jalapeño peppers, broccoli, and mushrooms fall under the umbrella of free food, those methods of preparation turn them into expensive foods. Free food aims to keep the calorie count as low as possible. Typically, free and almost-free foods are non-starchy vegetables. Free food only costs you up to 25 calories per serving. Almost-free foods contain 25–60 calories per cup. Usually, a serving amounts to one cup of these veggies chopped. These vegetables have such a low-calorie count per volume because they are higher in water and fiber than their starchy counterparts. They also have higher nutrition to calorie ratio, as they're packed with vitamins, minerals, and antioxidants that are good for you, but the weight for weight doesn't have as many calories as, say, potatoes. Think about it for a moment. At just 25 calories or less per cup, you can eat 10 cups of free-food vegetables for a mere 250 calories! Almost-free vegetables will cost you between 250 and 600 calories for the same amount. If that isn't a bargain, I don't know what is.

What about protein? Indeed, lean cuts of red meat, pork, poultry, and fish don't contain carbohydrates, but they do still contain calories. You see, carbs and protein cost four calories per gram while fat costs a whopping nine calories per gram. When you're filling up on free food, the idea is to keep your calories low but the volume high. Protein is dense and heavy; therefore, it costs more per weight than non-starchy vegetables. For example, one ounce of lean, skinless, uncooked chicken breast will cost you 34 calories. To put that into perspective, that's a piece of chicken breast roughly ⅓ to ¼ the size of a deck of playing cards. A whole cup of cherry tomatoes, on the other hand, is only 26.8 calories. See the calorie cost versus volume difference?

Okay, so the protein doesn't count, and starchy vegetables aren't on the list, but what about fruit?

Fruit is also packed with nutritious goodness and fiber, so it should count as free food, shouldn't it? Well, yes, fruit is good for you, but it's also pretty high in natural sugars. A single cup of blueberries takes 85 calories out of your daily allowance. That's 60 calories more per cup than the requirement for a food to be considered free. Even watermelon, with its water content so high, doesn't count as free food at 47 calories per cup.

THE BENEFITS OF FIBER OVER CARBS

The fiber-to-carbohydrate ratio is the game changer when it comes to free and almost-free foods. Carbohydrates translate into sugar when they are broken down during digestion. However, not all carbohydrates are created equal. Let me explain. Carbs are made up of sugars and fiber—at least most of them are. Each food has a total carbohydrate value and a net carb value. The net carb value is what counts toward the calorie value of a portion of food because that is the part of the total carbohydrate that is digested and influences your blood sugar level. The fiber part of the total carbohydrate value is indigestible and simply passes right through—not affecting your blood sugar at all. Why is this important?

Carbs can be divided into complex and simple carbs. All vegetables, even the starchy ones, contain complex carbohydrates while sugar and processed food typically contain simple carbohydrates. Simple carbs are those that have been processed, and they have heavily reduced fiber and nutrients. This means that they affect your blood sugar more and have more calories weight for weight than complex carbs.

Now, I've just said that even starchy vegetables contain complex carbohydrates and fiber, but the ratio with fiber to net carbs of starchy veggies is much lower than non-starchy vegetables. In a nutshell, the carbohydrates in non-starchy vegetables contain more fiber and less sugar while the carbs in starchy vegetables contain less fiber and more sugar. This makes starchy vegetables have more calories than non-starchy vegetables. Let me demonstrate what I mean.

Comparing simple carbs, non-starchy vegetables, and starchy vegetables:

Nutritional value per cup	Simple carbohydrate	Starchy vegetable	Non-starchy vegetable
Food item	Refined white sugar	White potatoes	Cherry tomatoes
Calories	774	103.5	26.8
Total carbohydrate	200 grams	23.6 grams	5.8
Fiber	0 grams	3.6 grams	1.8
Net carbohydrate	200 grams	20 grams	4

As you can see, when comparing white potatoes with cherry tomatoes:

- White potato fiber makes up only about 15% of the total carbohydrate while the net carb makes up around 85%.
- Cherry tomato fiber makes up roughly 32% of the total carbohydrate while the net carb makes up roughly 68%.

Fiber acts as a filler in foods. Your body cannot digest it, so it simply bulks out your food—making you feel full quicker and for longer after a meal or snack. Along with bulking out your food, it also slows down digestion. Carbohydrates containing less fiber, however, are less bulked out and digest quicker, allowing you to eat more calories per volume and leaving you feeling hungrier sooner.

PREPARATION IS KEY

When you go through the list of non-starchy vegetables in the next section, you will notice broccoli and mushrooms listed. Remember when I said that tempura fried broccoli and stuffed mushrooms won't count as free or almost-free foods? Considering they are listed, why aren't they free? Not only does the freeness of the food depend on the calorie content of the actual vegetable but it also depends greatly on how you prepare that vegetable.

When you add ingredients such as egg dip, flour, and bread crumbs for a coating, you are adding additional calories. Combine that with the oil that is soaked up during deep frying, and you have added a ton of calories which knocks the food right out of the free food park. Similarly with stuffing vegetables, you are adding a variety of other ingredients that up the calorie cost of the food.

How you prepare your free or almost-free veggies is vital to whether they maintain that free status. Does this mean you have to munch your way through raw vegetables for them to continue to be free? Not at all! You just need to use preparation methods that will keep the calorie content comparatively low.

Important Note: A serving of fresh vegetables is typically one cup chopped for most vegetables and two cups shredded for leafy green vegetables. However, when vegetables are cooked, the serving changes to half a cup because the volume gets smaller, but the nutrition stays the same.

▷ **Forget Frying**

Did you know that oil costs an incredible 135 calories per single tablespoon? You are dramatically increasing the calorie count of any food by adding fat or oil to your cooking process. Deep-frying vegetables in a coating allows that already carb-heavy coating layer to just soak up oil like a sponge. Even fries, which aren't coated, soak up oil on the outside. The amount of fat and calories you are adding to your diet by deep-frying any kind of food isn't worth it when there are various other delicious ways to prepare your food.

▷ **Roasting, Grilling, and Sautéing**

You can more easily control how much oil you use when you sauté, grill, or roast vegetables. However, these cooking methods do ramp up the calories and should probably only be used as preparation methods occasionally. You could use low-calorie cooking sprays to coat nonstick pans and grills for grilling and sautéing, but you are still adding a surprising number of calories to your low-calorie vegetables. Unfortunately, when roasting vegetables, you can't just give the pan a quick coat of nonstick spray. Your vegetables will dry out, so you need to toss them in a coating of oil to prevent that. The best way to ensure your free and almost-free vegetables stay that way is to forget about adding fat to the cooking process.

▷ Boiling and Steaming

Boiling and steaming non-starchy vegetables is the only way to ensure you don't add any calories to the serving you're eating. Boiling and steaming get a bit of a bad reputation because most people consider it to be a bland way of cooking food, but it doesn't have to be. You can still season your vegetables with herbs and spices to give them a delicious flavor. You don't have to stick to single portions of one type of steamed vegetable either. You would be surprised at the wide variety of warm, cooked salads available to keep you enjoying your veggies during the cold winter months. The only consideration to give boiling vegetables is that vital nutrients often leach out into the water they are being boiled in. This lowers their overall nutritional value.

▷ **Going Raw**

Eating the veggies you can eat raw is truly the best way to make sure you are getting the ultimate benefits as far as nutrition is concerned. Raw veggies maintain their nutrients, giving your body what it needs to be healthy. Now, you may think only a small selection of vegetables can be eaten raw, but you would be astounded at how many vegetables can be enjoyed raw when they're sliced, diced, or shredded into a salad. Using a variety of different vegetables in several different salads will help you avoid eating non-starchy vegetables from becoming boring. As they say, variety is the spice of life.

Important Note: Salad dressings for both raw and cooked salads will increase the calorie value of the salad. However, using reduced-calorie dressings and using them sparingly will help you keep the calorie increase as low as possible. I highly recommend a mix of lemon juice, a splash of vinegar and some fresh or dried herbs as a great addition to any plate of veggies or salad.

NON-STARCHY VEGETABLES

Well, with all this talk of non-starchy vegetables as free and almost-free options to fill up on, you're probably wondering what vegetables fall under the category of non-starchy. A good rule of thumb to use when considering whether a vegetable is starchy or not is to look at whether it grows underground or aboveground. Vegetables grown underground tend to be the plants' storage for sugars, so they have more starch in them. Why is that? Well, tuber plants don't give off seeds. Instead, new plants grow out of the tubers (or vegetable parts) underground. Plants that grow aboveground typically produce seeds to give rise to the next generation of plants. These seeds don't require all that extra starch to germinate and grow.

Here's a list of non-starchy vegetables to get you started on snacking and filling up on low-calorie foods:

❀ Amaranth leaves (Chinese spinach)

❀ Artichokes

❀ Asparagus

❀ Baby corn

✿ Bamboo shoots

✿ Beans (not legumes)

- Green beans
- Wax beans
- Italian beans

✿ Beets

✿ Broccoli

✿ Brussel sprouts

✿ Cabbage

- Red
- Green
- Bok choy/pak choi
- Chinese

✿ Carrots

✿ Cauliflower

✿ Celery

✿ Chayote (custard marrow)

✿ Coleslaw

- Packages with no dressing

✿ Cucumber

✿ Daikon (winter radish)

✿ Eggplant

✿ Fennel

✿ Hearts of palm

✿ Kale

✿ Kohlrabi

✿ Leeks

✿ Lettuce

- Green leaf
- Read leaf
- Romaine
- Iceberg
- Butter lettuce
- Little gem lettuce
- Mixed baby lettuce (Mesclun)
- Stem lettuce
- Speckled lettuce
- Coral lettuce (Lollo Rosso and Lollo Bionda)

✿ Mushrooms

✿ Okra

✿ Onions

✿ Peapods

- Sugar snap peas
- Snow peas

✿ Peppers (all types)

✿ Radishes

✿ Rutabaga

✿ Salad greens

- Arugula (rocket)
- Baby Spinach
- Baby spinach
- Beet greens
- Chicory
- Collard greens
- Dandelion
- Endive
- Escarole
- Mâche (field salad)

- Mustard greens
- Napa cabbage
- Oakleaf
- Radicchio
- Swiss chard
- Watercress

✿ Scallions

✿ Spinach

✿ Sprouts

- Alfalfa
- Chickpea
- Kidney bean sprouts
- Lentil sprouts
- Mung bean
- Pea sprouts
- Soybean

✿ Squash

- Crookneck
- Cushaw
- Spaghetti
- Summer

✿ Tomatoes

✿ Turnips

✿ Water chestnuts

✿ Zucchini

14

DAY 27: YOU'VE MADE IT! WHAT NEXT?

You've made it through the meal plan. You may have lost all of the weight you wanted to lose or at least some of it—depending on what your weight loss goals are. Once you've lost the weight, you can't let your guard down and allow poor eating habits to creep back in. This will lead to weight gain and a cycle of yo-yo dieting which is super unhealthy and can lead to ending up heavier than you were before you started the weight loss-weight gain cycle. You definitely don't want that.

I've given you all the tools and a great guideline for building a healthier, happier future for yourself. Once you've lost the weight, it's time to plan for healthy weight management moving forward. What does that mean?

MAINTAINING A HEALTHY WEIGHT

Maintaining a healthy weight requires different sources of motivation for different people. Here are some good tips to help you stay the course to a healthier, long-term lifestyle and maintain a healthy weight.

- **Keep Track:** It can be tempting to relax your grip on your new healthy eating habits after you've reached your goal weight. To help you keep an eye on your daily calorie intake, use a diet tracking app. There are various apps available that allow you to log what you eat, and they'll automatically tally up your calories and macros.
- **Set New Goals:** Some people need to constantly be working toward new goals. Once you've reached a healthy weight and achieved that goal, it may be time to start looking for your next goal. What would you like to achieve? Perhaps you want to work toward fitness goals to help maintain your weight and improve your cardiovascular fitness, flexibility, stamina, and range of motion as you get older.

- **Team Up With a Buddy:** This is a great idea when you are starting with your new, healthy lifestyle. Holding yourself accountable for developing new healthy habits can be difficult. After all, who's going to know if you cheat on your diet? You have someone else to help consistently hold you accountable when you work with a diet or fitness buddy. They have similar goals and will encourage you to keep up with your new eating habits when your motivation falters.

HEALTHY DIET MAINTENANCE TIPS

These tips come in handy while you're getting into the groove of your new healthy eating habits, but they are especially useful for keeping that healthy lifestyle going once you've lost weight. Try out some of these tips and tricks to help you keep the pounds off:

▷ **Drink Water**

There are many reasons we reach for food that have nothing to do with physical hunger. Some examples include stress, boredom, peer pressure because others are eating (eating is associated with socializing), and even dehydration. If you're feeling hungry shortly after a healthy meal, reach for a glass of water before grabbing a snack. Thirst can easily be confused with hunger, so you might just be thirsty.

▷ Drink Hot Beverages

If water isn't doing the trick, try drinking a hot beverage, but beware of reaching for high-calorie drinks like hot chocolate or a flavored cappuccino. You should also keep an eye on your caffeine intake. Beverages like tea or bone broth are lower in calories, and the heat of each sip will help make you feel full longer than a cold beverage.

▷ Pack In the Protein and Fiber

Protein takes longer to digest than carbohydrates, keeping your tummy feeling full for longer. You should also choose your carbs carefully. Whole foods and whole grains are rich in fiber which fills you up quickly and not only helps keep things regular but also doesn't digest which will also help keep you feeling full after a meal.

▷ Don't Keep Calorie-Rich Snacks on Hand

What's the easiest way to grab a calorie-laden snack? By keeping it on hand. Stock your fridge and cupboards with healthy snacks, like fruit and vegetables, and banish unhealthy snacks from your home. That way, you're forced to reach for a healthier option when you do have a snack attack.

▷ Stay Busy

Boredom is a notorious snack fiend. We are all tempted to munch when we have nothing else to do. You don't have to run yourself off your feet every minute of every day to avoid boredom snacking. Find something relaxing to do in your spare time that will help you keep your hands and mind busy while also reducing stress; coincidentally, this is another reason we reach for snacks when we're not really hungry.

▷ Retrain Your Taste Buds

Did you know that sugar is addictive? According to a study published on Researchgate.net, sugar is more addictive than cocaine. Rats were given a choice between intravenous cocaine and intensely sweet water with saccharin in it. A whopping 94% of the rats involved in the study chose the sweet water time and time again—even when their cocaine doses were upped (Lenoir et al., 2017). Cutting added sugar out of your diet means retraining your taste buds to become attuned to natural sugars which aren't as sweet. Fruit is packed with natural sweetness as well as fiber and vital nutrients. Once your taste buds and brain have been reconditioned to subtler, natural sweetness, those pesky sugar cravings should die down.

▷ **Prep Your Meals**

One of the easiest ways to allow your healthy eating habits to go out the window is not knowing what you're eating or not having time to prepare nutritious meals. Preparing meals in advance can help solve the problem of keeping your healthy diet on track. You can also control your portion sizes by cooking bulk meals and dividing them into correctly sized portions before sticking them into the freezer. You are essentially creating delicious, nutritious, and homemade microwave meals! Another way you can prepare meals ahead of time is to cook enough at one meal to allow you to enjoy the leftovers the next day.

By failing to prepare, you are preparing to fail.

— BENJAMIN FRANKLIN

▷ **Get Your Family to Join**

One of the best ways to keep you on the straight and narrow is to get your family to buy into a healthy diet. If you live on your own, it's relatively easy to ban junk food from your kitchen, but if you live with a spouse, it's not as simple. If you have kids, it's an even bigger battle because everybody knows how much kids love unhealthy food and snacks these days. Getting everyone to buy into a healthy diet makes your life a lot easier when it comes to meals as well.

You won't have to try to cook separate meals or separate meal ingredients for you and your family. What I mean by this is you won't have to take the extra time to cook separate healthier vegetables and whole grains for yourself while also preparing a less healthy meal for your family.

The second way it makes mealtimes easier is that you won't have to feel like the odd one out. It's not fun trying to ditch old habits and develop new ones when others around you aren't changing their habits. It's not going to be particularly fun if you have a side salad with your grilled chicken while your spouse and kids are digging into fried battered chicken and potatoes smothered in butter. Having everyone enjoying the same delicious, healthy food will prevent you from feeling left out at the dinner table.

▷ **Reduce Your Stress**

Stress can literally kill you, but it can also easily be the death of your healthy diet and lifestyle attempts. Stress can lead to emotional eating. Come on, be honest. How often do you crave and cave in to comfort food after a long and stressful day or week? It also leads to food cravings that may feel impossible to resist. That's not all. Stress also saps your motivation right out of you and makes preparing home-cooked meals seem daunting. This is where meal prep beforehand comes in super handy. Bringing down your stress levels will go a long way to maintaining a healthy diet for the long haul.

To reduce your stress, try the following:

- Getting regular exercise which produces

feel-good hormones in your body and improves your mood.

- Unplugging from the world from time to time by switching off your electronics and spending some "me time" doing something just for yourself
- Taking up new hobbies you enjoy that will help boost your mood
- Taking time to breathe with breathing exercises
- Getting outdoors where you can appreciate nature and get some fresh air
- Lighting scented candles or burning incense you like the smell of: Lavender is a great option for its calming effects.
- Get enough sleep: Your brain functions better and handles stress easier when it's not tired.

These are just a few suggestions. Find what works for you and indulge in it regularly. Managing your stress doesn't happen with a one-time indulgence—just like losing weight and keeping it off doesn't happen with a one-time diet. You need consistency for maintenance.

▷ **Get Your Body Moving**

Let's talk about exercise. Not only can exercise help you reduce your stress but it is also a vital component for a well-rounded, healthy lifestyle. When you combine diet and exercise, the health benefits are doubled. Do you know how people start to complain more and more about aches, pains, and stiffness as they age? Regular exercise will also help you reduce muscle mass loss and keep your muscles and joints flexible by maintaining your range of motion.

Now, when you think of exercise, what mental image pops up in your head? Does it involve sweating it out on the treadmill or spending hours at the gym? I thought it might be because that is the stereotypical idea many people have about exercise. However, that doesn't have to be the case—especially if you haven't been getting regular exercise for a while. Exercise can be as simple as walking. Walking is an effective form of exercise that gets your body moving and your heart rate up. Add some stretching or even some basic yoga to regular walks, and you have a recipe for success.

Nothing is impossible. The word, itself, says "I'm possible!"

— AUDREY HEPBURN

LET'S TALK SUPPLEMENTS

Various perimenopause symptoms are made worse because of nutritional deficiencies. Some of these deficiencies are a direct result of a deficiency in your diet. However, some deficiencies start cropping up because your body becomes less efficient at absorbing and using crucial vitamins and minerals as you age. It's worthwhile considering dietary supplements if you think you may have a mineral or vitamin deficiency.

Important Note: Always consult your physician before taking any supplements—even over-the-counter varieties. You could also consult a knowledgeable pharmacist, but your doctor is the only one who can give you a thorough once-over and tell you what you may need to take. Part of adopting a healthy lifestyle is always playing it safe. The health benefits you achieve aren't going to amount to much if you end up sabotaging your health in other aspects.

▷ Calcium

One of the problems with dwindling hormone levels throughout perimenopause and beyond is the potential for bone density loss. This makes getting enough calcium vitally important to maintain strong, healthy bones and minimize your risk of osteoporosis and fractures.

You need 1,000 mg of calcium per day under the age of 51.

You can get calcium from your diet, but if you find you just aren't hitting that sweet 1,000 mg sweet spot, consider a supplement.

▷ Flaxseed

Flaxseed is a natural dietary supplement that has two major benefits. Ground flax seeds make a fantastic addition to cooked breakfasts like oatmeal or smoothies, and the high fiber content makes it a great "filler" to keep you feeling full between meals. The second benefit is that flax seeds are rich in lignans which could help regulate your fluctuating hormones.

▷ Ginseng

Ginseng is often associated with revitalized energy and a reinvigorated libido, but that's not all. It can help you deal with stress more effectively which acts as a mood-lifting pick-me-up and makes dealing with perimenopausal symptoms at least a little easier.

▷ Soy

Before you write soy off as a meat supplement for vegetarians and vegans, hear me out. Soy may just be the secret to helping you tame hot flashes. It contains natural estrogen-like chemicals which could just help relieve mild hot flashes in peri-menopausal women.

▷ Vitamin D

Vitamin D is also fondly called the sunshine vitamin. It's made in your skin when your skin is exposed to direct sunlight—another reason to go for a walk outdoors! Vitamin D is vital for your bone health, as calcium cannot be absorbed without it. You should be aiming for around 600 IU, or an international unit, per day. Once you hit the age of 71 you'll need about 800 IU per day. Yes, you're going to hit the big number 70, and you're going to be enjoying the quality of life because of the healthy changes you make to your diet and lifestyle today. If you can't get enough sun exposure to produce the required amount of vitamin D, you may want to consider taking a supplement.

15

SECRETS TO A FLATTER TUMMY AND BEATING BLOAT

If there is one thing that is the bane of pretty much every single woman's existence, it's belly fat. I'm not talking about that dangerous visceral fat surrounding your organs inside your abdomen. I'm talking about the subcutaneous fat that gives your belly that little jiggle.

The diet plan and advice I've given you so far has been designed to help you lose overall body fat to slim down and become healthier, but what about that stubborn belly fat? Sit tight because I'm about to give you five additional tips to trim down belly fat for a flatter stomach. Let's get started, so you can start working on a flatter tummy today.

CURB THE "ADULT" BEVERAGES AND CAFFEINE

Your body is made up of mostly water, so it stands to reason that it needs lots of it. Alcoholic beverages, on the other hand, dehydrate your body and pause fat loss. You see, your body sees alcohol as a toxin, and its reaction is to try to get rid of that toxin by flushing it out of your system. Your liver prioritizes getting rid of alcohol over anything else. Have you ever noticed that you need to visit the bathroom more frequently after a drink or two? You guessed it: That's your body registering the alcohol and trying to get rid of it. Another downside of drinking adult beverages is that it bloats your face. Who wants to look in the mirror to see a puffy face staring back? Not only that but it can also cause bloating in your midsection. If you enjoy going out with your girlfriends for a drink, try to curb your alcohol intake or opt for a nonalcoholic mocktail instead. Just be aware of the sugar content of the mixers used.

Alcohol isn't the only culprit of tummy bloat. Coffee and tea may have the same effect—especially if you're sensitive to the ingredients. That's not to say you have to have major adverse reactions to the caffeine and ingredients in coffee and tea. You could have some low-key reactions you don't take notice of at first, such as bloating. It does this because—just like you get a caffeine buzz—your digestive system may do the same and become over excited and bloated as a result.

Along with curbing your alcohol and caffeine intake, you should try to increase how much water you drink. Water doesn't just flush alcohol out of your system, but it also flushes other toxins out as well—detoxifying your body. For a great-tasting, water-detox drink, try adding some mint, lemon, or cucumber to your water to boost that detox effect. If you want to reach for a warm beverage, try switching to green or even chamomile tea if green isn't your "cup of tea." Better yet, drink one of these teas before you exercise to boost your fat-burning efforts. Another trick to try is adding ginger to your tea or making ginger tea. Ginger will help calm your gastrointestinal system to reduce unsightly and uncomfortable bloating.

STRESS LESS

Let's talk about stress. Everybody knows it's really bad for your overall health, but we don't seem to make enough of an effort to reduce it. In today's world, stress may even be viewed as a badge of honor. After all, the more stressed you are, the busier you are, and being busy is often associated with success. The problem with stress is that it's also associated with weight gain (especially around your tummy area). You can thank the stress hormone cortisol for this as I've previously mentioned. However, stress can also irritate your digestive system, causing indigestion and bloating.

Exercise is the closest you can get to a "miracle pill." It helps combat a variety of health risks, gets your stress under control, and burns body fat. Aerobic exercise releases feel-good hormones which reduce stress, but you don't have to stop there. Sweating it out on the treadmill isn't your only option. Walking is gentle and effective for raising your heart rate and releasing those hormones. You can also try incorporating light yoga into your weekly, or even daily, routine. Yoga helps you focus on your breathing and becoming in tune with your body while you're transitioning from pose to pose. Taking your mind off the worries of the world and focusing on yourself is a great way to let go of your daily stress load and lower anxiety.

SLEEP IS UNDERRATED

Have you ever heard of the phrase, "I'll sleep when I'm dead"? Well, let me tell you, sleep may not outright kill you but lack of it does amp up your stress levels which can put you at greater risk of health conditions. Sleep is vitally important for both your body and your mind; it's downtime that helps your mind rest and your body recover. Yes, your body needs to recover from energy expenditure and stresses placed on it during a busy day. It's when your muscles recover from strain, your cells regenerate, and your energy levels are replenished. Getting enough sleep also allows you to lose weight and regulate your weight better. How does the simple act of sleep help you lose weight?

- You have more energy which allows you to exercise more intensely or for a longer period of time.
- Your appetite could increase. Combine constantly having the munchies with poor decision-making by a tired mind, and you could not only eat more but make unhealthy food choices more easily.
- You could experience a rise in cortisol which

not only prompts your body to store more
fat but to store it around your tummy.

How much an individual needs to sleep per night
varies from one person to the next, since we're all
unique, and our bodies operate differently from
everyone else. However, you should try to aim for
around seven to eight hours of sleep per night.

LAY OFF THE SALT

Do you like salty foods or adding salt to your meals?
You may want to consider curbing your love of salt.
Salt causes water retention which not only reflects
an incorrect number on the bathroom scale but also
contributes to bloat. It could also go the other way. If
you're eating too much salt, your body could try to
flush it out of your system by getting rid of water,
and you could end up being dehydrated. Who knew
salt could have such effects on your body? If you
want to lay off the salt but still enjoy delicious food,
try adding herbs and spices while cooking instead.
You still get tons of flavor without the added salt and
the side effects that come with it. On the other hand,
if you do genuinely have an intense salt craving, it
could be an indication of a deficiency in your diet,

and you may want to pop in at your doctor's office to make sure you are getting all the proper vitamins and minerals you need.

EXERCISE THAT TUMMY LEAN

I've mentioned some tips for getting rid of belly fat, but what about once that fat is gone? Once you have a flat tummy, you're not going to be completely satisfied with just a soft flat tummy. You're going to want a toned tummy—even if you don't have or want a six-pack in the end. What you need is to incorporate exercises that target your abs. These exercises may not target belly fat, but they will reveal toned abs once that belly fat melts away. Another benefit of strong abs is they form part of your core muscles which help stabilize your body and your spine. A strong core means there's less pressure on your skeletal structure and reduces your risk of injury. Some of the best ab exercises include:

- Sit-ups
- Crunches
- Planks
- Leg raises

These are just a few of the many ab exercises out there. To motivate yourself to work on your abs, you must pick exercises that are comfortable and enjoyable for you. You also need to make sure you get your form correct. A poor form makes an exercise less effective and can lead to injury.

SHOW YOUR LIVER SOME LOVE

Your liver is an underrated organ that performs a multitude of functions to keep your body healthy. It's where fat is broken down for weight loss, where toxins are removed from your bloodstream, and it helps regulate your hormones. When you neglect your liver, it can cause weight gain and bloat. An unhealthy liver cannot process sugars and toxins properly which leads to a buildup of fat stores in various parts of your body. An unhealthy liver may also cause bloating; again, it's unable to process substances in your body properly which could cause fluid to build up in your midsection. As a perimenopausal woman battling her fluctuating hormones and the middle-aged spread, why wouldn't you want to look after your liver? Here are some tips for showing your liver some love.

▷ Avoid Alcohol

Not only does alcohol have the potential to cause bloating but it also has negative effects on your liver. As I've just explained, your body sees alcohol as a toxin, and your liver jumps into action to rid your body of it. The more alcohol you consume, the more stress you are putting on your liver. This can lead to developing fatty liver which leads to weight gain or even cirrhosis of your liver tissue (which is when your liver cells start to die). To avoid damage to your liver, step back from alcoholic drinks and opt for water or even mocktails instead.

▷ Start Sweating

While there are various reasons for fatty liver disease, two of the most common causes are consuming too much alcohol and being overweight. Now, just because you're overweight doesn't mean you automatically have a fatty liver, but carrying around too much weight can lead to it. Fatty liver disease makes your liver less efficient at doing its many jobs. Doing exercise routines that get your heart rate up helps reduce the amount of fatty buildup in your liver. This improves liver health and function.

CONCLUSION

Perimenopause is an inevitable part of any woman's life, but it doesn't have to signal the end of your life. You don't have to resign yourself to being ruled by out-of-whack hormones and suffer the middle-aged spread. You can take control back and change your body and quality of life. It may seem like an impossible mission when you first think about it, but that couldn't be further from the truth. Yes, you are going to have to put in the work, and it isn't going to be a simple walk in the park, but your health and happiness are worth it.

I came very close to accepting my perimenopausal fate because, "That's just the way it is, right?" I'm here to tell you how it doesn't have to be that way.

I look better now than I have ever looked in my life. It's been five years of hard work in the making amid crazy perimenopausal hormonal changes. My saggy butt is long gone and so is my flabby tummy. I have a six-pack for the first time in my life! The most important lesson I have learned is that food is your mood and the best medicine. It is so simple and yet so difficult to achieve. This is especially true when we, as women, believe in fad diets, don't know anything about carbs, and have a tendency toward emotional eating. Most of us spend a huge part of our lives not really having an understanding of or grasp about nutrition. Add to that the hormonal storm perimenopause brings with it, and we think it's game over.

To truly change, I had to accept myself. I had to learn that I needed to change my mindset; instead of changing my body because I hated it, I had to change my body because I loved it. I learned an awful lot by trial and error. I learned to make a balanced diet—calculated according to my TDEE which is part of my lifestyle. Introducing new habits was hard, and it seemed to take forever! Once I had the healthy diet down pat, I focused on building muscle and strength, but that is a topic for another book though.

Everything starts with good food… and a plan.

I am continuing to work toward my body goals every day. It is my new lifestyle now—despite many challenges. I set my goals and work toward them slowly but surely. I hope you will take the information and guidance I've provided you with to make the same changes I did. I have never looked back, and my future looks so much brighter than I could ever have expected in those first perimenopausal years. I took control, and you can do the same thing. What are you waiting for? To start seeing the changes you want in your life tomorrow, you need to start building new habits today.

THANK YOU!

Thank you for choosing this book!

I truly hope it has been a very useful resource to you on your journey through perimenopausal weight loss and lifestyle change. If this is the case, please take two minutes to review it on Amazon and recommend it to others. I will be honored to read your feedback in order to create more valuable content in the future. By leaving your review, you will help a small independent publisher make a big difference to many women across the world.

All you need to do is click on the Amazon review link below and share your thoughts with others.

https://www.amazon.com/review/create-review/?asin=

A sentence or two is perfect, or just a star rating if you are really short of time! If you have two more free minutes, take a photo or video of yourself with the book and post it straight on Amazon. I cannot wait to see your feedback!

If you choose to subscribe to my newsletter, I am very much looking forward to hearing from you personally soon!

You can find all the details on the next page.

Sarah

xo

YOUR FREE GIFT

Thank you so much for purchasing this book!

Scan the QR code or visit our webpage via the link
below to receive a FREE mini e-book:

"7 EASY STEPS to Reduce Hormonal Bloating Fast

+

5 Day Quick Fix Meal Plan"

www.perimenopausematters.com

REFERENCES

Adkins, P. (2018, March 11). [Article about not regretting getting older]. Medium. https://medium. com/@pixienoire/dont-ever-regret-growing-older- it-s-a-privilege-denied-to-many-b0fc71e76b6a

American Heart Association Editorial Staff. (2015). *Portion size versus serving size.* American Heart Asso- ciation.https://www.heart.org/en/healthy-living/ healthy-eating/eat-smart/nutrition-basics/portion- size-versus-serving-size

Audrey Hepburn Quotes. (n.d.). BrainyQuote.com. Retrieved October 13, 2021, from BrainyQuote.com Web site: https://www.brainyquote.com/ quotes/audrey_hepburn_413479

Banana & almond butter toast. (n.d.). Health. https://www.health.com/recipes/banana-almond- butter-toast

Basaraba, S. (2020, January 24). *Common age-related diseases and conditions.* Verywell Health.

https://www.verywellhealth.com/age-related-diseases-2223996

Basaraba, S. (2020, January 24). *Common age-related diseases and conditions*. Verywell Health. https://www.verywellhealth.com/age-related-diseases-2223996

Benjamin Franklin Quotes. (n.d.). BrainyQuote.com. Retrieved October 12, 2021, from BrainyQuote.com Web site: https://www.brainyquote.com/quotes/benjamin_franklin_138217

Bleeding after menopause: Is it normal? (n.d.). Mayo Clinic. https://www.mayoclinic.org/diseases-conditions/menopause/expert-answers/bleeding-after-menopause/faq-20058396

Blueberry oatmeal porridge with honey for breakfast. (2021, August 11). Recipe Garden. https://recipe-garden.com/blueberry-oatmeal-porridge/

Bryan, L. (2019, March 29). *Blueberry smoothie.* Downshiftology. https://downshiftology.-com/recipes/blueberry-smoothie/

Bush, A. (2020, October 5). *Vegetable omelette.* Olive Magazine. https://www.olivemagazine.com/recipes/healthy/vegetable-omelette/

Camacho, P. (2009). *Estrogen replacement therapy for osteoporosis.* Endocrine Web. https://www.endocrineweb.com/conditions/osteoporosis/estrogenreplacement-therapy-osteoporosis

Camarcho, P. (2009). *Estrogen replacement therapy for osteoporosis.* Endocrine Web. https://www.endocrineweb.com/conditions/osteoporosis/estrogenreplacement-therapy-osteoporosis

Casner, C. (2017, May). *Mediterranean chickpea quinoa bowl.* Eating Well. https://www.eatingwell.com/recipe/258195/mediterranean-chickpeaquinoa-bowl/

Cervoni, B. (2015, January 26). *Load up on nonstarchy vegetables.* Verywell Health. https://www.verywellhealth.com/load-up-on-nonstarchy-vegetables-1087520

Charles Kettering Quotes. (n.d.). BrainyQuote.com.

https://www.brainyquote.com/
quotes/charles_kettering_121333

Chelsea. (2020, March 3). *Yogurt bowl*. Chelsea's
Messy Apron. https://www.chelseasmessyapron.-
com/top-10-favorite-ways-top-yogurt-bowl/

Cherney, K. (2017, October 10). *Weight gain and
menopause*. Healthline. https://www.healthline.-
com/health/menopause/weight-gain

Cherney, K. (2017, October 10). *Weight gain and
menopause.* Healthline. https://www.healthline.-
com/health/menopause/weight-gain

Cherry tomatoes, red, ripe, raw, year round average.
(n.d.). Eat This Much. https://www.eatthismuch.-
com/food/nutrition/cherry-tomatoes,1221840/

Chertoff, J. (2020, March 30). *Which is better for your
health: Walking or running?* Healthline.
https://www.healthline.com/health/walking-vs-
running

Chertoff, J. (2020, March 30). *Which is better for your
health: Walking or running.* Healthline.

https://www.healthline.com/health/walking-vs-running

Clancy, J. (2017, September/October). *Berry-almond smoothie bowl*. Eating Well. https://www.eatingwell.com/recipe/259665/berry-almond-smoothie-bowl/

Coleman, E. (n.d.) *How many calories are in 1 oz of meat and poultry?* Livestrong. https://www.livestrong.com/article/314196-how-many-calories-are-in-1-oz-of-meat-poultry/

Connors, C. (2018, March 23). *7 Principles to Develop Toughness and Build the Life You Want to Live*. Thrive Global. https://thriveglobal.com/stories/7-principles-to-develop-toughness-and-build-the-life-you-want-to-live/

Detoxing your liver: Fact versus fiction. (n.d.). Johns Hopkins Medicine. https://www.hopkinsmedicine.org/health/wellness-and-prevention/detoxing-your-liver-fact-versus-fiction

Di Lorenzo, P. M., Chen, J.-Y., Rosen, A. M., & Roussin, A. T. (2020). Tastant. *Encyclopedia of Neuro-*

science, 4014–4019. https://doi.org/10.1007/978-3-540-29678-2_5888

Dickerson, L. M., Mazyck, P. J., & Hunter, M. H. (2003). Premenstrual Syndrome. *American Family Physician, 67*(8), 1743–1752. https://www.aaf-p.org/afp/2003/0415/p1743.html

Dickerson, L. M., Mazyck, P. J., & Hunter, M. H. (2003). *Premenstrual syndrome.* American Family Physician. https://www.aafp.org/afp/2003/0415/p1743.html

Eating lots of carbs, sugar may raise risk of cognitive impairment. (2012, October 16). Mayo Clinic study finds. Mayo Clinic. https://newsnetwork.mayoclin-ic.org/discussion/eating-lots-of-carbs-sugar-may-raise-risk-of-cognitive-impairment-mayo-clinic-study-finds/

Emily. (2014, June 19). *Loaded Mediterranean veggie sandwich.* Layers Of Happiness. https://www.layersofhappiness.com/loaded-mediterranean-veggie-sandwich/

Estrogen's effects on the female body. (n.d.) Johns

Hopkins Medicine. https://www.hopkinsmedi-
cine.org/health/conditions-and-diseases/estrogens-
effects-on-the-female-body

Estrogen's effects on the female body. (n.d.) Johns
Hopkins Medicine. https://www.hopkinsmedi-
cine.org/health/conditions-and-diseases/estrogens-
effects-on-the-female-body

Filtness, K. (n.d.). *How to improve your liver health
through exercise.* Nature's Best. https://www.natures-
best.co.uk/our-blog/how-to-improve-your-liver-
health-through-exercise/

Freeman, K. (2019, September 22). *Carrot sticks with
hummus.* The Healthy Eating Hub.
https://healthyeatinghub.com.au/carrot-sticks-
with-hummus/

Galan, N. (2018, May 17). *Can estrogen levels affect
weight gain?* Medical News Today.
https://www.medicalnewstoday.com/articles/321837

Galan, N. (2018, May 17). *Can estrogen levels affect
weight gain?* Medical News Today.
https://www.medicalnewstoday.com/articles/321837

Gallagher, A., & Gallagher, J. (n.d.). *Chimichurri cauliflower steaks*. Inspired Taste. https://www.in-spiredtaste.net/48013/chimichurri-cauliflower-steaks/

Gallagher, A., & Gallagher, J. (n.d.). *Guilt-free garlic parmesan zucchini noodles pasta*. Inspired Taste. https://www.inspiredtaste.net/29992/garlic-zucchini-pasta-recipe/

Gallagher, A., & Gallagher, J. (n.d.). *Lentil soup with lemon and turmeric*. Inspired Taste. https://www.in-spiredtaste.net/40400/lentil-soup/

Gallagher, A., & Gallagher, J. (n.d.). *Roasted veggie tacos with creamy cilantro sauce.* Inspired Taste. https://www.inspiredtaste.net/30196/roasted-veggie-tacos/

George Eliot Quotes. (n.d.). BrainyQuote.com. https://www.brainyquote.com/quotes/george_eliot_161679

Global Organics Staff. (2016, March 29). *4 categories of organic product labels*. Global Organics. https://www.global-organics.com/post.php?

s=2016-03-29-4-categories-of-organic-product-labels

Hagen, E. (2018, July 30). *10 hormones responsible for weight gain in women.* Vivify Interactive Health. https://vivifyintegrativehealth.com/blogs/10-hormones-responsible-for-weight-gain-in-women

Hagen, E. (2018, July 30). *10 hormones responsible for weight gain in women.* Vivify Integrative Health. https://vivifyintegrativehealth.com/blogs/10-hormones-responsible-for-weight-gain-in-women

Harmon, K. (2012, October 24). *How slight sleep deprivation could add extra pounds.* Scientific American. https://www.scientificamerican.com/article/sleep-deprivation-obesity/

Hazell, A. (2018, December 4). *BMR Formula (basal metabolic rate).* The Calculator Site. https://www.thecalculatorsite.com/articles/health/bmr-formula.php

Healthy Women Editors. (2015, May 13). *The truth about menopause and weight gain.* Healthy WomenOrganization. https://www.healthywomen.org/your-health/menopause-aging-well/truth-about-menopause-and-weight-gain

Hosterman, J. F. (2015, May 13). *The truth about menopause and weight gain*. Healthy Women Organization. https://www.healthywomen.org/your-health/menopause-aging-well/truth-about-menopause-and-weight-gain

How alcohol affects your appearance. (2021). Drinkaware. https://www.drinkaware.co.uk/facts/health-effects-of-alcohol/appearance/how-alcohol-affects-your-appearance

How alcohol affects your appearance. (2021). Drinkaware. https://www.scientificamerican.com/article/sleep-deprivation-obesity/

How much physical activity do adults need? (2020, October 7). Centers for Disease Control and Prevention [CDC]. https://www.cdc.gov/physicalactivity/basics/adults/index.htm

How to improve your liver health through exercise. (n.d.) Nature's Best. https://www.naturesbest.co.uk/our-blog/how-to-improve-your-liver-health-through-exercise/

Improve your liver function to boost metabolism. (n.d.). The Chiropracti Associates. https://www.chiroassoc.net/blog/2017/10/24/why-you-need-a-healthy-liver-for-metabolism

Johns, A. L. (2020). *30 Days of Inspirational Quotes for Weight Loss*. Lose Weight By Eating. https://loseweightbyeating.com/inspirational-quotes-for-weight-loss/

Johnson, S. (2021, January 27). *What are the possible causes of vaginal dryness*? Medical News Today. https://www.medicalnewstoday.com/articles/321615

Johnson, S. (2021, January 27). *What are the possible causes of vaginal dryness?*. Medical News Today. https://www.medicalnewstoday.com/articles/321615

Johnston, K. (2020, August 19). *Greek yogurt & fresh berries*. The Kitchen Magpie. https://www.thekitchenmagpie.com/greek-yogurt-fresh-berries/

Joyce Meyer. (n.d.). AZQuotes.com. https://www.azquotes.com/quote/448594

Koch, A. (2017, January 12). *Postit memo post it notes memory isolated notes.* Pixabay. https://pixabay.com/illustrations/postit-memo-post-it-notes-memory-1975188/

Laseter, E. (2018, April). *How to make the ultimate healthy breakfast smoothie*. Cooking Light. https://www.cookinglight.com/recipes/healthy-breakfast-smoothie

Laughlin-Tommaso, S. (n.d.) *Bleeding after menopause: Is it normal?* Mayo Clinic. https://www.mayoclinic.org/diseases-conditions/menopause/expert-answers/bleeding-after-menopause/faq-20058396

Lenoir, M., Serre, F., Cantin, L., & Ahmed, S. H. (2007). Intense Sweetness Surpasses Cocaine Reward. *PLOS ONE*, *2*(8), e698. https://doi.org/10.1371/journal.pone.0000698

Lenoir, M., Serre, F., Cantin, L., & Ahmed, S. H. (2007). *Intense Sweetness Surpasses Cocaine Reward*.

PLOS ONE, 2(8), e698. https://doi.org/10.1371/journal.pone.0000698

Lindsay. (2014, July 10). *Simple poached egg and avocado toast.* Pinch Of Yum. https://pinchofyum.com/simple-poached-egg-avocado-toast

Living on F-factor: Vegetables, the free food. (2019, June 12). F-Factor. https://www.ffactor.com/living-ffactor-vegetables-free-food/

Mayo Clinic Staff. (2019). *Perimenopause.* Mayo Clinic. https://www.mayoclinic.org/diseases-conditions/perimenopause/symptoms-causes/syc-20354666

Menopause causes. (2020, October 14). Web MD. https://www.webmd.com/menopause/guide/menopause-causes

Menopause causes. (n.d.) Web MD. https://www.webmd.com/menopause/guide/menopause-causes

Menopause, Perimenopause and post menopause. (2019, December 24). Cleveland Clinic. https://my.cleve-landclinic.org/health/diseases/15224-menopause-perimenopause-and-postmenopause

Menopause, Perimenopause and post menopause. (2019, December 24). Cleveland Clinic. https://my.cleve-landclinic.org/health/diseases/15224-menopause-perimenopause-and-postmenopause

Meyer, H. (2018, June). *No-cook black bean salad.* Eating Well. https://www.eatingwell.-com/recipe/265885/no-cook-black-bean-salad/

Minimalist Baker. (2017, October 28). *1-pot pumpkin yellow curry.* Minimalist Baker. https://minimalistbaker.com/1-pot-pumpkin-yellow-curry/

Mullins, B. (2021, August 28). *Cinnamon raisin oatmeal.* Eating Bird Food. https://www.eatingbird-food.com/cinnamon-raisin-oatmeal/

Okman-Kilic, T. (2015). Estrogen Deficiency and Osteoporosis. In *www.intechopen.com.* IntechOpen. https://www.intechopen.com/chapters/48016

Okman-Kilic, T. (2015). *Estrogen deficiency and osteo-*

porosis. IntechOpen. https://www.intechopen.-com/chapters/48016

Pass It On. (n.d.). *Dedication: Pass It On*. Pass It On. https://www.passiton.com/inspirational-quotes/7470-if-you-really-want-to-do-something-youll-find

Peeke, P. (2007, May 15). *Fit to Live: The 5-Point Plan to be Lean, Strong, and Fearless for Life*. Harmony/Rodale Books.
Perimenopause. (n.d.) Johns Hopkins Medicine. https://www.hopkinsmedicine.org/health/conditions-and-diseases/perimenopause

Perimenopause: Rocky road to menopause. (2020, April 14). Harvard Health Publishing. https://www.health.harvard.edu/womens-health/perimenopause-rocky-road-to-menopause

Petre, A. (2017, January 30). *5 ways restricting calories can be harmful.* Healthline. https://www.healthline.-com/nutrition/calorie-restriction-risks

Portion size versus serving size. (2015). American Heart Association. https://www.heart.org/en/healthy-living/healthy-eating/eat-smart/nutrition-basics/portion-size-versus-serving-size

Preserve your muscle mass. (2016, February 19). Harvard Health Publishing, Harvard medical School. https://www.health.harvard.edu/staying-healthy/preserve-your-muscle-mass

Printable PMS symptom tracker. (n.d.). Free Printable Medical Forms. https://www.freeprintablemedical-forms.com/preview/PMS_Symptom_Tracker

Pullen, C. (2017, June 6). *7 ways sleep can help you lose weight.* Healthline. https://www.healthline.com/nu-trition/sleep-and-weight-loss

Raidrsgal. (n.d.). *Herbed cheese and tomato sandwich.* Spark People. https://recipes.sparkpeople.-com/recipe-detail.asp?recipe=654824

Rodriguez, A. (2019, October 18). *Apple and peanut butter sandwich)gluten-free, vegan snack).* The Butter Half. https://www.thebutterhalf.com/apple-peanut-butter-sandwich-gluten-free-vegan-snack/

Roskelley, A. (2021, January 3). *Celery and peanut*

butter with calories and macros. Health Beet Organization. https://healthbeet.org/celery-and-peanut-butter-with-calories-and-macros/

Smith, H. (2018, July 23). *5 drinks you should avoid if you want a flat stomach.* Insider. https://www.insider.com/drinks-to-avoid-if-you-want-flat-stomach-2018-7

Stanton, B. (2020). *Starch 101: Resistant starch plus keto-friendly starch alternatives.* Carb Manager. https://www.carbmanager.com/article/xtqygheaaci-achjm/what-is-starch-and-why-is-it-bad-for-keto/

Stevens, K. (2012, November 12). *Easy vegetarian chili recipe (vegan chili!).* The Endless Meal. https://www.theendlessmeal.com/easy-vegetarian-chili-recipe/

Sugar, white, granulated sugar. (n.d.). Eat This Much. https://www.eatthismuch.com/food/nutrition/sugar,4644/

The dangers of visceral fat. (2016, May 11). Epic Wellness. https://www.epicwellnessvt.com/the-dangers-of-visceral-fat/

Thorpe, M. (2017, May 29). *10 solid reasons why yo-yo dieting is bad for you*. Healthline. https://www.health-line.com/nutrition/yo-yo-dieting

Waehner, P. (2020, December 3). *Talk test and monitoring exercise intensity*. Verywell Fit. https://www.verywellfit.com/talk-test-fitness-term-1231121

Wharton, W., E. Gleason, C., Sandra, O., M. Carlsson, C., & Asthana, S. (2012). Neurobiological Underpinnings of the Estrogen - Mood Relationship. *Current Psychiatry Reviews*, *8*(3), 247–256. https://doi.org/10.2174/157340012800792957

White potatoes, flesh and skin, raw. (n.d.). Eat This Much. https://www.eatthismuch.com/food/nutrition/white-potatoes,2093/

Why fiber makes weight loss easier. (n.d.). F-Factor. https://www.ffactor.com/what-is-f-factor/why-fiber/

Williams, N. I., Reed, J. L., Leidy, H. J., Legro, R. S., & De Souza, M. J. (2010). Estrogen and progesterone exposure is reduced in response to energy deficiency in women aged 25–40 years. *Human Reproduction (Oxford, England)*, *25*(9), 2328–2339. https://doi.org/10.1093/humrep/deq172

Your body's reaction to yo-yo diets explained in pictures. (n.d.) Web MD. https://www.webmd.com/diet/ss/slideshow-diet-yo-yo-diet-effect

Ingram Content Group UK Ltd.
Milton Keynes UK
UKHW021312010523
421053UK00018B/349